A DOCTOR'S ADVICE TO KEEP YOU OUT OF HIS OFFICE

To order additional copies of
"A DOCTOR'S ADVICE TO KEEP YOU
OUT OF HIS OFFICE"
call 616-243-8326 or
email ajubert@sbcglobal.net

A DOCTOR'S ADVICE TO KEEP YOU OUT OF HIS OFFICE

Eight FREE Prescriptions ...Better Than Any Pill... That Will Help You...

- ■ Supercharge Your Immune System
- ■ Avoid Disease
- ■ Enjoy Peak Health and Energy, and
- ■ Add Years to Your Life

ANDRÉ V. JUBERT, M.D., FACS

HOPE

Hamblin's Outreach Publishing Enterprises

Tecumseh, Michigan 49286

This book was
Edited by Ken McFarland
Cover designed by Bill Howison
Electronic makeup by Jeanne Knowlan
Typeset: Bookman 11/14

PRINTED IN U.S.A.

03   1

ISBN 0-9742729-0-6

Dedication

To my wife, children, and grandchildren

About the Author

Iwas born in Fort-de-France, Martinique, French Antilles. I came to the United States of America in 1958 and attended Emmanuel Missionary College, now Andrews University, in Berrien Springs, Michigan. I graduated from Andrews in 1961 with a major in biology and a minor in chemistry. I earned my medical degree from Howard University School of Medicine in 1966.

My first contact with the book *The Ministry of Healing,* by Ellen G. White, occurred while a pre-medical student at Andrews. My interest in the healing art led me, on my own, to read the book from cover to cover. This was not for a course or curriculum requirement.

The duties of the Christian physician outlined in *The Ministry of Healing* indelibly impressed me and influenced my practice of medicine and surgery from the outset in 1973 when I went into practice. To quote two statements: "The physician has precious opportunities for directing his patients to the promises of God's word. . . . Let him study the word of God diligently, that he may be familiar with its promises. . . . Never should he neglect to direct the minds of his patients to Christ, the Chief Physician" (p. 121).

"Knowing the Lord Jesus, it is the privilege of the Christian practitioner by prayer to invite His presence in the sick room. Before performing a critical operation, let the physician ask for the aid of the Great Physician. Let him assure the suffering one that God can bring him safely through the ordeal, that in all times of distress He is a sure refuge for those who trust in Him. The physician who cannot do this loses case after case that otherwise might have been saved" (p. 118).

These two paragraphs are just samples of the book that served to mold my mind in my formative years and helped formulate my philosophy of practice: The physician has no inherent healing powers in his hands; all healing comes from God; he is only an instrument in the hands of the Great Physician; he must remain submitted to Christ.

This philosophy has served me well over the past twenty-nine years as a surgical oncologist in Grand Rapids, Michigan, where my patients know me as the praying surgeon.

After graduating from medical school, I did a general surgery residency at St. Mary's Mercy Medical Center in Grand Rapids, Michigan, then spent two years of fellowship at the University of Texas M.D. Anderson Cancer Center in Houston, Texas. I returned to St. Mary's in 1973 and started their outpatient oncology clinic. I am now in private practice.

I am married to the former Bernice ("Bernie") Reaves. We have two adult daughters and two grandchildren.

Acknowledgments

Several pioneers have succeeded in establishing lifestyle centers in various sections of this country and abroad, based on the instructions given by Ellen G. White. I have borrowed heavily from their publications, sometimes using their basic outlines.

Special thanks go to the late Vernon W. Foster, M.D., for the autographed copy of his book, *Newstart*, given to me on January 26, 1989 during my first visit to Weimar Institute and to the institute itself in Weimar, California, for additional information.

I was privileged three years ago to spend a week at the Black Hills Health and Education Center at Hermosa, South Dakota. Thanks to Pastor Louie Torres and his wife Carol, then director of the center, for providing a copy of *Wellness to Fitness*, by Melvin Beltz, M.D., along with copies of dozens of typewritten pages on their health program. They were a tremendous help to me and helped solidify a new direction in my medical practice. Thanks also to Glenn Kerr, M.D., then medical director of the health program at Black Hills, for helpful tips.

Health pamphlets from Wildwood Lifestyle Center and Hospital, Wildwood, Georgia; Uchee Pines Institute, Seale, Alabama; and Lifestyle Center of America, Sulfur, Oklahoma, have also been appreciated.

A one-day clinic observation with clients at the Battle Creek Lifestyle Center, Battle Creek, Michigan, was also very helpful.

Although used by permission and properly annotated, it is proper, I believe, to acknowledge use of numerous quotations directly or, at times, indirectly, from Dr. Neil Nedley's book, *Proof Positive*.

To Rabbi Albert Lewis, retired spiritual leader of Temple Emanuel in Grand Rapids, Michigan—a long-time friend and now, writer, teacher, and counselor—I shall ever remain grateful. His literary critique and guidance have provided much added clarity to this work.

Last but not least, thank you to my wife, Bernie, for putting up with me for thirty-seven years of marriage, but especially for patiently enduring hours of "non-attention" to her during this writing, completed while maintaining a full-time surgical practice.

Finally, thanks to God for His infinite mercy and grace!

Contents

Foreword

To heal the human body is an act of skill and wisdom. To heal the body and the soul is the highest calling any physician or caring person can have. Such a person sees himself as an instrument of God and truly understands God's command to "seek mercy, do justly, and walk humbly with your God." A person who lives in this way is also a true partner with God. His words, hands, and heart are guided by the Ultimate Power.

Dr. Andre Jubert is such a person. As a devout Seventh-day Adventist, Andre is committed to more than healing—he is devoted to the very prevention of disease, whether it is physical or emotional. His reputation in the medical community is that of a physician who willingly prays with, advocates for, and does everything with the skills that God has given him to address the wholeness of the person before him.

A Doctor's Advice to Keep You Out of His Office is Andre's synthesizing of Seventh-day Adventist health and medical insights with contemporary research and knowledge. To read and truly follow *A Doctor's Advice* is to choose a life course infused with the love, caring, and nurturing God wants for all of His people.

I am proud to call Andre my friend and one of the physicians of my soul. As you read this book, you will find yourself ready to reflect on your lifestyle and choices—and to understand ever more profoundly that God wants all of us to be healthy. But the choice is ours. Reading and internalizing the wisdom of this book is an excellent beginning.

Dr. Albert Micah Lewis, Rabbi
The Aquinas Emeritus College
Grand Rapids, Michigan

Preface

Another book on preventing disease through lifestyle?

Let us first establish what this book is not. It is not a book to promote the use of "naturally grown" or "organically grown" vitamins. It is not a book on the benefits of "natural" supplements. It is not promoting the use of essential "organically extracted" oils or herbs or herbal teas. It is not for treating specific diseases by natural means.

The purpose of this work is not to provide new information, but to help disseminate "old" but very relevant information. As a physician, I have studied health counsels and instructions on prevention written in the late 1800s and early 1900s by Ellen G. White and directed to the Seventh-day Adventist Church as custodian, but counsels and instructions whose benefits were meant, I believe, to be trans-denominational and trans-cultural. These counsels have resulted in a relatively small denomination being able to maintain and operate health institutions, food stores, and restaurants around the world.

One of the outstanding contributions of the instructions given by Ellen G. White is the recognition that it is part of religious duty to care for the body temple. Churches, therefore, are to be involved in health education both inside and outside their borders, stressing prevention of disease. In the light of recent scientific discoveries, I am convinced that if those preventive measures had been more widely known, believed, and followed, the health of our population would be vastly improved and the cost of medical care would be a fraction of what it is today. The emphasis of our health system in this country for the past 100 years would have been on prevention, not on the cure of illnesses.

My burden, therefore, is to place this information in more and different hands. People in varied echelons of society have begun to take control of their health. The time seems ripe. A great interest exists in diet and exercise and a wholistic approach to health care. I am also greatly anxious to have as many of my fellow physicians as possible examine this information as I have and formulate their own conclusion about incorporating the principles into their practice. I believe it would make a difference in the health of their patients.

The following statement was made almost a century ago: "Pure air, sunlight, abstemiousness, rest, exercise, proper diet, the use of water, trust in divine power—these are the true remedies."[1]

This rather interesting statement has withstood the test of time, taking into consideration who made it and when it was made. The above principles are termed the "Eight Natural Remedies," or the "Eight Natural Laws of Health." They emphasize prevention of disease, an "ounce of which is better than a pound of cure." To be of benefit, however, they require knowledge of them and their faithful daily practice or application to our lives, as well as knowledge of the workings of our bodies. And for those who have taken the time to study and practice them, they have proven effective.

A few months ago, a young man in his early twenties came to me on referral from his physician, for evaluation and treatment of an advanced melanoma of his thigh. There were large lymph nodes in his groin. It was then that the thought occurred to me to write these remedies in prescription form—steps to be followed on a daily basis—in the hope of strengthening his immune system. To date, he remains free of disease, strong, and lifting weight. He is completing his education while working on a part-time basis to help defray his expenses.

These prescription forms have now become part of my office offerings to my patients, who, for the most part, express surprise at the simplicity of these remedies. They cost no money—just the commitment of time and effort on their part.

This book is the outgrowth of that experience, which began over a year ago now. Each chapter is launched with a quotation that applies to the natural remedy under consideration (the last two are preceded with a Bible verse, as well). Then, an outline of the section is provided. The section discussing each Natural Remedy then begins with a prescription.

I have taken the liberty of changing the order in which these principles appear in *The Ministry of Healing*, to present the natural remedies instead in the order of their importance, as concerns their necessity to sustain life. We can live but a few minutes without air. It will be days before our bodies dehydrate and we die without water. And we can go on for months without food, as witnessed by "hunger protests" for various causes in this country and abroad, for example.

Ellen G. White was a Bible student. Her book *The Desire of Ages* has been acclaimed as one of the best expositions on the life of Jesus Christ ever written. It is therefore not surprising that the eight natural remedies she presents are all Bible-based.

Almost all, in fact, are found in the first two chapters of Genesis—proof, I believe, that they are necessary to maintain our state of well-being. They were given before the fall and hence, before sickness and death.

It is my hope that all who read this book will commit time and effort to put these eight steps into practice in their daily lives, and will thereby feel a resurgence of vitality, clarity of mind, and strength of body.

Note:

1. Ellen G. White, *The Ministry of Healing* (Mountain View, Calif.: Pacific Press, 1905), p. 127.

Chapter 1
The History Behind the Eight Prescriptions

Focus: *The Ministry of Healing*—a book written by Ellen G. White and published in 1905. Who was Ellen G. White? And what was the state of medical practice in 1905?

Ellen G. White

The following is an excerpt from her own biographical sketch:

"I was born at Gorham, Maine, November 26, 1827. My parents, Robert and Eunice Harmon, were for many years residents of this State. In early life they became earnest and devoted members of the Methodist Episcopal Church. In that Church they held prominent connection, and labored for the conversion of sinners, and to build up the cause of God, for a period of forty years. During this time they had the joy of seeing their children, eight in number, all converted and gathered into the fold of Christ. . .

"While I was but a child, my parents removed from Gorham to Portland, Maine. Here, at the age of 9 years, an accident happened to me which was to affect my whole life. In company with my twin sister and one of our schoolmates, I was crossing a common in the city of Portland, when a girl, about 13 years of age, becoming angry at some trifle, followed us, threatening to strike us. Our parents had taught us never to contend with anyone, but if we were in danger of being abused or injured, to hasten home at once. We were doing this with all speed, but the girl followed us as rapidly, with a stone in her hand. I turned my head to see how far she was behind me, and as I did so, she threw the stone, and it hit me on the nose. I was stunned by the blow and fell senseless to the ground.

"When consciousness returned, I found myself in a merchant's store; my garments were covered with blood, which was pouring from my nose and streaming over the floor."

Ellen attempted to walk home but soon became faint and dizzy. "My twin sister and my schoolmate carried me home. . . . My mother said that I noticed nothing, but lay in a stupor for three weeks."[1]

Everyone, except her mother, thought she was going to die. Ellen's curiosity was aroused as she gained consciousness and heard comments about her appearance. "I asked for a looking glass, and was shocked, upon gazing into it, at the change of my appearance. Every feature of my face seemed changed."[2] As she gained strength, she attempted on three occasions to resume her classes but could not. She finally abandoned all prospects of a formal education three years after the accident at the age of 12—basically at a third-grade level.

She obviously did not die. At the age of 17 she married James White, a minister and one of the founding fathers of the Seventh-day Adventist Church, and lived until the age of 87. She died on July 16, 1915.

Ellen G. White wrote voluminously on such varied topics as education and child-rearing; the life, death, and resurrection of Jesus Christ; His work of intercession in heaven; end-time events in relation to the conflict between good and evil; the Old Testament patriarchs, prophets, and kings; the acts of the apostles and the early Christian Church; and the second coming of Christ. She gave both personal, individualized messages and corporate, generalized counsels to her church—the Seventh-day Adventist Church.

As a physician, I was most impressed with her numberless articles on health. In addition to *The Ministry of Healing*, written in 1905, her manuscripts have been compiled into several books: *Counsels on Health, Counsels on Diet and Foods, Temperance,* and *Medical Ministry.* She placed great emphasis on lifestyle and disease prevention and on the relationship between observance of natural laws and well-being. I was also impressed with her concepts as to the cause of disease, and the best means of alleviating sickness—from proper diet and the use of water, to adequate exposure to sunshine and fresh air and ventilation of the sick room. Her explanation of the rapport between the mental, social, physical, and spiritual dimensions of the human body set forth concepts of wholistic medicine far ahead of the medical science practiced at the time. I was impressed with her counsels concerning the close relationship that should exist between the health ministry and the gospel ministry in the church. She counseled that, following the example of Jesus, health ministry should always precede the preaching ministry. Indeed, one needs only to take a cursory look at the four gospels to realize that Jesus did more healing than preaching. She was a great Bible student.

She helped guide the burgeoning educational system of the Seventh-day Adventist Church, especially at times of crises, both here and abroad. She spent several years in Australia and played a vital role in the location and the mission of Loma Linda University in Loma Linda, California.[3]

How could she have gained the knowledge to counsel in matters of health, especially—even if this knowledge had been available—with less than a third-grade education? The Seventh-day Adventist Church, based on Joel 2:28 and 29, has always believed she was inspired of God. As a Bible-believing Christian physician, I fully concur.

So these instructions as just mentioned, if indeed given by inspiration, transcend denominational boundaries and were intended for the health benefits of the whole world.

Indeed, a noteworthy national broadcaster, appreciatively calling her "the little lady," recommended her writings to America.[4]

The state of medical practice in 1905

Some pioneer work had been done in health reform, going back to the birth of this country. "Dr. Benjamin Rush, one of the signers of the American Declaration of Independence in 1776, wrote a pamphlet in 1785 entitled 'Inquiry Into the Effects of Ardent Spirits.' In it, he appealed to heads of Government and to ministers of the Gospel, to arouse and aid him with all the weight they possessed in Society, from the dignity and usefulness of their sacred office, to save fellowmen from being destroyed by the great destroyer of their lives and soul."[5]

January 10, 1826 saw the organization of the American Temperance Society in Boston, Massachusetts. In less than a decade, "the Society grew to about 5,000 local chapters, and more than a million members."[6] However, by the middle of the nineteenth century, the initial activity and success of the temperance movement had greatly abated. Local societies, to a large degree, had ceased to function.

The earliest consideration of vegetarianism seems to have been in England in 1809, through a book written by William Lambe, M.D. Fifty years later, the American Vegetarian Society was first organized.

The summer of 1777 saw the birth of hydrotherapy. William Wright, a physician from the island of Jamaica, was on board a ship bound for Liverpool. In treating a case of typhus fever which ended fatally, he became infected and was very ill.

"After a series of self prescriptions including gentle vomit, followed by a decoction of tamarands, and at bed time an opiate joined with antimonial wine, and a drachm of Peruvian, back every hour for six hours successively with an occasional glass of port wine, and feeling no better, he was perplexed. He noted, however, that when he went on deck he experienced decided relief—the colder the air, the better."[7]

"This circumstance," he reported, "and the failure of every means I had tried, encouraged me to put in practice on myself what I had often wished to try on others, in fevers similar to my own."[8] In desperate hope, he had three buckets of sea water thrown over his naked body. Though "the shock was great, he felt immediate relief. He repeated the treatment when the fever reappeared a few hours later, and did it twice the following day. . . . Every symptom vanished, but to prevent a relapse, he used the cold bath twice the third day," he recorded in his diary.[9]

"Soon, another passenger was taken down with the same fever, and at his urgent request, Dr. Wright ventured to give him the same treatment, with the same gratifying results."[10]

But this is pretty harsh treatment. It is much preferable for one shaking with a high fever and chills to climb under a warm blanket and take a pill and drink a warm drink than to be immersed in a bath of ice cold water or have ice-cold sea water from the middle of the North Atlantic poured on him. It is understandable that "cold and hot" water as a remedy would not be popular. Instead, there was heavy reliance on drugs for the treatment of diseases. Very little attention was paid to the prevention of disease.

So even though there had been trends and movements since the birth of this country in the direction of natural remedies, these concepts which Ellen G. White advanced were not common knowledge in 1905 and certainly not routinely practiced, even among health professionals.

John Janvier Black, M.D., writing five years earlier in 1900, states: "Learned professors had their own ideas and opinions, and these ideas and opinions were generally derived from someone equally emphatic who had preceded them, probably amplified from time to time as light gradually began to show itself on the medical horizon. Yet, most of their ideas and opinions had not fact, scientific or otherwise, for their basis, but an absolutely empirical origin; in other words, true science had not yet dawned upon medical practice and medical thought."[11]

As for diet, Dr. Black states: "Little was said about it, and less was taught concerning it in the medical schools. All, or nearly all, at that time, believed, empirically believed, in antiphlogistin system of treatment (treatment designed to reduce inflammation, understood at that time, as bleeding, and the use of salts and antimony); and almost every sick man, or wounded man, or crazy man, for that matter, was put on a diet as near bread and water as possible."[12]

In contrast, writes Ellen G. White, "Our bodies are built up from the food we eat. There is a constant breaking down of the tissues of the body; every movement of every organ involves waste, and this waste is repaired from our food."[13]

Also, "Grains, fruits, nuts, and vegetables constitute the diet chosen for us by our Creator. These foods, prepared in as simple and natural a manner as possible, are the most healthful and nourishing. They impart . . . strength, . . . power of endurance, and . . . vigor of intellect."[14]

Notes:

1. Ellen G. White, *Testimonies for the Church*, vol. 1 (Mountain View, Calif.: Pacific Press Publishing Association, 1948), pp. 9, 10.

2. Ibid., p. 10.
3. Herbert E. Douglass, *Messenger of the Lord: The Prophetic Ministry of Ellen G.White* (Nampa, Idaho: Pacific Press Publishing Association, 1998), p. 356.
4. Paul Harvey News, 1969.
5. D. E. Robinson, *The Story of Our Health Message* (Nashville: Southern Publishing Association, 1943), p. 38.
6. Ibid., p. 41.
7. James Currie, M.D., *Medical Reports on the Effects of Cold and Warm Water as a Remedy in Fever and Other Diseases,* vol. 1, pp. 1-4 (London: Printed for T. Cadell and W. Davis, 1805), as quoted by D.E. Robinson, *The Story of Our Health Message* (Nashville: Southern Publishing Association, 1943), p. 29.
8. Ibid.
9. Ibid.
10. Ibid.
11. John Janvier Black, M.D., *Forty Years in the Medical Profession* (Philadelphia: J. B. Lippincott Co., 1900), p. 126.
12. Ibid., p. 187, as quoted in D. E. Robinson, *The Story of Our Health Message*, p. 19.
13. Ellen G. White, *The Ministry of Healing* (Mountain View, Calif.: Pacific Press Publishing Association, 1905), p. 295.
14. Ibid., p. 296.

Chapter 2

"In order to have good blood, we must breathe well. Full, deep inspirations of pure air, which fill the lungs with oxygen, purify the blood. They impart to it a bright color and send it, a life-giving current, to every part of the body . . .

"The lungs should be allowed the greatest freedom possible. Their capacity is developed by free action; it diminishes if they are cramped and compressed. Hence the ill effects of the practice so common, especially in sedentary pursuits, of stooping at one's work. In this position it is impossible to breathe deeply. Superficial breathing soon becomes a habit, and the lungs lose their power to expand. A similar effect is produced by tight lacing. Sufficient room is not given to the lower part of the chest; the abdominal muscles, which were designed to aid in breathing, do not have full play, and the lungs are restricted in their action . . .

"Thus an insufficient supply of oxygen is received."—Ellen G. White, *The Ministry of Healing*, pp. 272, 273.

Air

In this section we will discuss:
- How our heart and lungs work.
- Nature's ecological system.
- Cigarette smoking and its effects on our body.
- Proper breathing technique and its benefits.
- The best time to exercise—and why.

■ Brief spiritual lesson to be derived from breathing.

Prescription No. 1:

Air

Every half hour, outside or in front of an open window, take three deep breaths, inhaling through the nose and exhaling through the mouth. (The abdomen should push out during inhalation—allowing the diaphragm to come way down, filling the lower segments of the lungs with air—and push in during exhalation.)

Pure, fresh air is essential for life. At creation, after God removed darkness on the first day by creating light, we are told, "God made the firmament" (Genesis 1:7)—the life-giving atmosphere encircling the earth.

This life-giving atmosphere, in order to benefit us, must penetrate into every cell of our bodies. For this, God created the respiratory and circulatory systems in our bodies. The mouth, the nose, the pharynx, the larynx, the trachea, and the lungs, make up the respiratory system. The circulatory system is comprised of the heart and the blood vessels. Arteries carry oxygenated blood from the heart; veins carry blood loaded with carbon dioxide to the heart. From the heart, the blood goes to the lungs to be reoxygenated and return to the heart.

The more intact we keep these systems, the better they function to provide air to our individual cells. Proper posture and breathing techniques are extremely important.

Air contains approximately 20 percent oxygen, slightly less than 80 percent nitrogen, and 1 percent carbon dioxide, with other trace elements. Nitrogen, used by plants to make protein, serves as a diluting agent for the oxygen we breathe.

Breathing carries oxygen from the air into our lungs, where, as simply put as possible, tiny breathing units called alveoli are in contact with tiny circulatory units called capillaries. There the exchange of oxygen and carbon dioxide is made. (We will leave surfactant, alveolar inflation, capillary hydrostatic pressure, etc. to the pulmonologist and the medical and surgical intensivist.) The oxygen is carried to every cell in our bodies by red blood cells. We have billions of these oxygen-carrying red blood cells in our bloodstream. In fact, red blood cells live for 120 days and must be continually replaced. The body produces about 2.5 million every second.

Improper breathing, as well as a reduction in the number of red blood cells in our bloodstream (anemia), results in ill health.

This exchange of oxygen and carbon dioxide points to the design of a Master Ecologist. God created the world with perfect recycling principles and laws. Plants use the nitrogen, as mentioned earlier, and then produce oxygen. People and animals breathe in this oxygen and breathe out carbon dioxide. Plants, in turn, use the carbon dioxide. So plant life supports animal life, and animal life supports plant life. Ecology did not start with man!

God cares about us and about the earth He created for us. He expects us to take good care of it, as well as of our bodies. We are where we are today with the ozone layer; global warming; air pollution; pollution of lakes, rivers, and seas; and our state of health (respiratory problems, etc.,) because we failed to pay attention to and obey those recycling principles God gave us (finding ways to use the by-products of industry instead of discarding them.)

The several million tons of pollutants released into the air each year damage our body tissues and decrease their ability to use oxygen. We may not be able to do much about the tons of pollutants released by industry, but there is one pollutant produced by individual habits which all of us can influence. Cigarette smoke, whether directly in the smoker, or indirectly by second-hand smoking, affects all.

Cigarette smoke contains more than forty cancer-causing chemicals, which result in several cancers at different sites in the body—the mouth, including the lips; the tongue; the cheeks; as well as the pharynx, the larynx, and the esophagus; the lungs; the pancreas; the kidneys; and the urinary bladder. Whereas 70 percent of these cancers could be prevented by not smoking, the five-year cure, across the board, in treating these cancers caused by cigarette smoking is 3 percent to 10 percent. The exception is cancer of the urinary bladder, which causes bleeding and is diagnosed early, with a 50 percent five-year cure rate.

In addition to the forty cancer-causing chemicals, cigarette smoke contains over 4,000 other chemicals, many of which are poisonous, toxic, or damaging to genes.[1]

Almost as bad as its cancer-causing effect on the lungs and other tissues is the effect of cigarette smoking on the protective mechanism of the air passages and the pulmonary alveoli, causing bronchitis and emphysema.

It has always been known that cigarette smoking is related to development of asthma in adults. Several recent studies document that second-hand smoking is one of the main causes of asthma in children.

So we owe it to ourselves, as a society, to stop smoking and its effects on our health and the health of our children.

But even in the absence of cigarette smoking, most of us could improve the amount of oxygen we breathe in. For the most part, we do not have good body posture, and we do not use our abdominal muscles to breathe, thus making our breathing too shallow.

The complex muscle-motor system required for breathing starts with the neck muscles and includes the chest muscles, the diaphragm, and the muscles of the anterior abdominal wall. The upper chest, the lower chest (diaphragm), and the abdomen are all necessary for proper breathing, but the most important is abdominal breathing. This allows the diaphragm to come way down, thus filling the lower lungs with oxygen.

What are the results of improper breathing? With improper breathing, our bodies, especially our brains, lack oxygen. We become mentally sluggish, fatigued, depressed, and eventually confused. With lack of oxygen, we become anemic; we have low creativity, poor memory, poor concentration, and poor quality of sleep.

"Failure to breathe properly robs us in most areas of life. It dulls such fine points of mental activity as will power, discernment, and judgment. It also affects our feelings. We are prone to develop such negative feelings as anger, low self-esteem, false guilt and pain. In short, by not using" this first natural remedy, "we rob ourselves of the joy of living."[2]

Improving one's breathing is a relatively easy procedure. However, it requires awareness, concentration, diligence, and perseverance to reverse the patterns established over many years. But the reward is worth the effort.

Begin today.

So if you are indoors, at home, or at the job sitting down at a computer desk, and you realize your mind is getting sluggish, it is because you have probably been slumped down, rebreathing the same carbon dioxide-filled air over and over. Get up, find an open window, or better yet, if you can, go outside, stand up straight with shoulders back, and inhale through your nose, using your lower chest and anterior abdominal wall muscles to suck in the air deeply and exhale through your mouth. Repeat this three or four times. You will feel more alert and will become more productive.

As a principle, we should exercise regularly in the outdoors or in a well-ventilated area, preferably in the morning when the highest concentration of negative ions is in the air. It is also a good practice to crack open your window to sleep. Fresh air purifies the blood and electrifies the body.

Fresh air is chemically different than recirculated indoor air. The life-giving oxygen molecule is negatively charged or "negatively ionized." Among the benefits of negatively charged fresh air are: "improved sense of well being, decreased anxiety, lowered resting heart rate, decreased survival of bacteria and viruses in the air, improved learning in mammals."[3]

"Good quality negatively ionized air is found in abundance in natural outdoor environment, especially around evergreen trees, beach surf, or after a thunderstorm. . . . On the other hand, negatively ionized air is destroyed by wind storms (dust storms), tobacco smoke, city smog, and other pollutants."[4]

So what spiritual lesson can we draw from this first prescription?

In talking with Nicodemus, when Jesus wanted to explain the working of the Holy Spirit in our lives, He compared it to air, or wind. He said in John 3:8: "The wind bloweth where it listeth, and thou hearest the sound thereof but canst not see whence it cometh, and wither it goeth: so is everyone that is born of the Spirit."

Pure air is invisible. It is colorless, odorless, and tasteless. We can only see the effect of its oxygen content in the faces of healthy people.

In another spiritual dimension, commenting on the life of Enoch, Ellen G. White tells us that Enoch "lived in the very atmosphere of heaven . . . to him prayer was as the breath of the soul."[5]

Wesley L Duewel, in *Mighty Prevailing Prayer*, quotes O. Hallesby, who states: "A child of God can grieve Jesus in no worse way than to neglect prayer. . . . Many neglect prayer to such an extent that their spiritual life gradually dies out."[6]

The parallel is obvious. Physically, we can live but a few minutes without breathing!

Notes:

1. Kent County Health Department, State of Michigan, *In Every Puff* (Center for Substance Abuse Prevention, 2/01).
2. Vernon W. Foster, M.D., *NewStart!* (Santa Barbara: Woodbridge Press Publishing Company, 1988), p. 145.
3. Baldwin, B.E., "Why Is Fresh Air Fresh?" *The Journal of Health and Healing*, 11(4): 26, 27, as quoted in Neil Nedley, M.D., *Proof Positive: How to Reliably Combat Disease and Achieve Optimal Health through Nutrition and Lifestyle* (Ardmore, Oklahoma: Quality Books, Inc., 1998), p. 500.
4. Neil Nedley, M.D., *Proof Positive*, pp. 500, 501.
5. Ellen G. White, *Patriachs and Prophets* (Mountain View, Calif.: Pacific Press Publishing Association, 1958), p. 85.
6. Wesley L. Duewel, *Mighty Prevailing Prayer* (Grand Rapids, Michigan: Zondervan Publishing House, 1990), p. 30.

Chapter 3

"In health and in sickness, pure water is one of heaven's choicest blessings. Its proper use promotes health. It is the beverage which God provided to quench the thirst of animals and man. Drunk freely, it helps to supply the necessities of the system and assists nature to resist disease. The external application of water is one of the easiest and most satisfactory ways of regulating the circulation of the blood. A cold or cool bath is an excellent tonic. Warm baths open the pores and thus aid in the elimination of impurities. Both warm and neutral baths soothe the nerves and equalize the circulation."—Ellen G. White, *The Ministry of Healing*, p. 237.

Water

In this section we will discuss:

- The prevalence of water in nature and in the human body.
- Dehydration—What is it?
- The symptoms of dehydration.
- Our need of water.
- A recommended schedule to drink eight glasses of water a day.
- Three additional general rules for drinking water.
- The advantages of the bath—historical setting.
- Hydrotherapy and other methods.
- Brief spiritual lesson from water.

Prescription No. 2:

Water

Use plenty of water both inside and outside the body.

Inside: Drink six to eight glasses of water daily.

Outside: Take a hot and cold shower (alternating hot and cold two to three times) twice a day for two weeks, then once a day thereafter. Finish with cold water in the morning and with hot water in the evening, especially before going to bed. When unable to shower, a "cold-mitten" friction can be helpful. (Take a cold, damp washcloth and briskly rub all accessible body parts until the skin becomes pink or a warm glow is felt all over.)

As stated in chapter 1, the birth of hydrotherapy was probably in 1777.

However, in the beginning, God made provision for the sustaining waters to be available for the rest of His creation. He knew water was the perfect substance to meet the needs of what He had planned for this planet.

Water is virtually everywhere and in everything. It covers more than three-fourths of the earth's surface and is the major component of the food we eat. Lettuce, for example, is 96 percent water—even more than fruit juice, which is 90 percent water. Even the foods we consider dry contain some water. Crackers have 5 percent water, bread, 36 percent, nuts and dry cereals, 2 percent to 3 percent, and dried fruits, 25 percent.

Water is the number one component of the human body. Body parts, however, vary in their contents: the brain is 70 percent to 85 percent water; muscles, 75 percent; while bones are 50 percent water. Water is involved in every body function. It quenches thirst, aids digestion, and relieves constipation. It cools the body during exercise. It carries and distributes nutrients to every cell and cooperates with the organs to flush out wastes. Water is a solvent and dilutes toxins. It lubricates joints and works as a shock absorber. It is an active part of blood, lymph, mucus, and digestive juices. It helps regulate body temperature.

Thirst lets us know that our bodies need water. A little more water taken each day, other than just for the satisfaction of thirst, is very essential to meet the needs of the body and to keep normal the body temperature. In fact, if one waits until one is thirsty to drink, one has waited too long for proper body function.

Dehydration is known as the loss of water from the body, and many have a tendency toward this. We lose water every day, not only from our kidneys, and our lungs, as we breathe, but also from tears and perspiration.

What are some of the effects of dehydration? Because the body is made up of such a high percentage of water, one would expect the effects of dehydration to be generalized or systemic. And indeed, they are.

Starting with the brain with its fifteen billion to forty billion cells, dehydration causes decreased mental alertness, depression, and irritability. With dehydration comes a concentration of body fluids, a change in mineral balance, decreased oxygenation, and thickening or greater viscosity of the blood.

The following chart, used by permission, from the teaching files at Black Hills Health and Education Center, shows that the severity of symptoms corresponds to the degree of dehydration or the percent of fluid loss:

Percent of Body Fluid Loss	Symptoms
2%	Increased thirst and decreased appetite, strong, concentrated urine
5%	Flushed skin, impatience, weariness, sleepiness, nausea, decreased urine output
7%	Tingling, stumbling, headaches, confusion, increased pulse, respiration, and elevated temperature
10%	Spastic muscle, delirium, cyanosis, indistinct speech
15%	Shriveled, numb skin, inability to swallow, deafness, no urine output
20%	Death[1]

On the other end of the scale, excess intake of water can lead to water intoxication, with dilution of body salts.

Many, if not most of us, however, don't drink enough water. Some have not drunk water in years. They say it makes them nauseated. But our bodies need six to eight glasses of water each day, and more in hot weather and after exercise. This is in addition to the water we get from food.

How to get eight glasses of water a day? As you get up in the morning, drink two glasses; in mid-morning, two glasses; in mid-afternoon, two glasses; and after supper, two glasses. You may find it easier to drink warm water, especially early in the morning.

Some other points: As a general rule . . .

■ We should avoid drinking too hot or too cold. Water is absorbed more quickly if it is tepid or at room temperature.

■ "Any sugar added to the drink retards and hinders replenishment. So, commercial preparations, which contain 5% glucose, would significantly retard replacement of fluid lost during exercise in the heat."[2]

■ We should avoid drinking water with meals. This slows down digestion by diluting digestive juices and can cause indigestion. To get the most benefit from the food we eat, we should drink thirty to sixty minutes before meals, and one to two hours afterward. Speaking from experience, I can state that it can become a matter of habit. One can reeducate oneself. Have no drinks on your table at mealtime. It may be hard at first, but with determination, it can be done.

What are some benefits of drinking water? Fewer headaches, better-regulated blood pressure, less bowel constipation, more energy, less muscular pain after exercise, less chance of kidney stones, fewer kidney and urinary bladder infections, and a clearer mind.

Obviously, just as drinking water cleanses the internal organs of the body, so water can keep the outside of the body clean. The Bible indicates that God expects personal cleanliness in body, clothing, and living quarters, as in the heart. In Exodus 19:10, as God was preparing to speak to Moses and the children of Israel on Mount Sinai after they left Egypt, He told Moses, "Go to the people and consecrate them today and tomorrow, and let them wash their clothes." When Aaron and his sons went into the Tabernacle to officiate, they were to "wash their hands and their feet in water, lest they died" (Exodus 30:19-21). Before they could put on their priestly garments and be consecrated, "Moses brought Aaron and his sons and washed them with water" (Leviticus 8:6). We read in Numbers 8:21: "And the Levites purified themselves and washed their clothes; then Aaron presented them before the Lord."

These verses of Scripture confirm the saying, "Cleanliness is next to Godliness"! It is interesting that this concept is not just Judeo-Christian. "Mohammed ordered his people to bathe before each of their five daily prayers."[3]

The value of water in preventing disease was recognized by ancient peoples. Baths were used then to a far greater extent than in modern times. "The Greeks regarded the bath as a very essential means of securing physical health. . . . The Romans also made a luxury of the bath. . . . Interestingly, during the Dark Ages in Europe, the bath was unknown among the masses. Michelet, a noteworthy historian, tells us that, in his opinion, 'this accounted for the terrible plagues and pestilences of that period.' . . . Remarkable of the Dark Ages (538-1798), was the absence of the Word of God, the Bible, from the common people. And so, they could not appreciate and make use of one of God's greatest gifts"[4]—pure water, His second natural remedy—to prevent disease.

And indeed, water can be used for treatment through the various forms of hydrotherapy—pool, tub bath, shower, hot-and-cold, steam, steam inhalation, ice massage for joints and muscle pain, and fomentation, which is the application of moist heat through a pad or towel to areas of the body.

One of the major factors driving up the cost of medicine today is the price of prescription drugs.

About 100 years after William Wright had cold sea water poured on his naked body on board ship on his way to Liverpool and cured his cases of Typhus fever, as mentioned in chapter 1,[5] Wilhelm Wintermitz of Vienna, Austria, and J. H. Kellogg, one of his pupils from America, established hydrotherapy as a scientifically applied and effective medicine. On his return home, in Battle Creek, Michigan, Dr. Kellogg expanded the use of hydrotherapy. "A core of nurses was trained in its skillful application with remarkable results. People came from all over to the Battle Creek Sanitarium."[6] Hydrotherapy is used today in lifestyle health centers in this country and abroad as a major therapy, as opposed to the use of drugs, and is still very effective. Why is it not as popular today?

The answer is that we are living in a drug-oriented society. People want a pill—a quick fix. For the most part, they don't want to take the time that natural processes require to get better. Especially since, for natural processes to work, a radical change, or what at first seems like a radical change in personal conduct and habit, must take place.

But the question we must ask is: Are drugs really the answer? All drugs have side effects. I often remark to my patients that if aspirin were discovered today, the FDA would most likely not approve it as an over-the-counter drug.

The natural remedies have no side effects. Water, hot or cold, as medicine, is inexpensive and readily available to all at home. Used with common sense, it has no hidden, unknown side effects (too hot a fomentation can burn the skin, of course, but common sense should guard against that! And diabetics, with decreased sensation in the lower extremities, should be supervised). However, its proper use requires time and effort on the part of the individual patient. One reason water is so useful is that it can hold and transport tremendous amounts of heat. Heat causes dilatation, or enlargement of blood vessels, to the area where it is applied, supplying it with a generous number of germ-fighting white blood cells, nutrients, and oxygen. Cold, on the other hand, constricts blood vessels, squeezing out or preventing the inflow of blood; thus preventing swelling and more tissue damage after injury, for example. So as a general rule, cold is indicated immediately after injury and for the next twenty-four to thirty-six hours. Heat is usually indicated for more chronic, long-term problems.

Is there a spiritual lesson to be drawn from Prescription No. 2?

At creation, "The Spirit of God moved upon the

face of the waters" (Genesis 1:2). Not only was God about to do something marvelous with water for our physical bodies, but Jesus says that He has "living water for anyone who is thirsty" (John 7:10). He promises all, as He did the woman of Samaria, that the water He gives to those who ask of Him will be in them a "well springing up into everlasting life" (John 4:14). Ellen G. White, commenting on this verse in the chapter "At Jacob's well," in her book, *The Desire of Ages*, states: "This woman represents the working of a practical faith in Christ. . . . He who drinks of the living water becomes a fountain of life. The receiver becomes a giver. The grace of Christ in the soul is like a spring in the desert, welling up to refresh all, and making those who are ready to perish eager to drink of the water of life."[7]

Jesus alone can satisfy the thirsty soul. In His Sermon on the Mount, He said, "Blessed are they which hunger and thirst after righteousness, for they shall be filled" (Matthew 5:6).

So with your two glasses of water, as you drink next time, allow your mind to dwell on the love of God, who created that water—and let your soul be filled with the superabundant grace He has provided for all.

Notes:

1. Vernon W. Foster, M.D., *NewStart* (Santa Barbara: Woodbridge Press, 1988), p. 91.
2. Melvin Beltz, M.D., *Wellness to Fitness* (Hermosa, South Dakota: Black Hills Health and Education Center, 1991), p. 2.
3. *History of Bathing*, Teaching Files on Hydrotherapy (Hermosa. South Dakota: Black Hills Health and Education Center), used by permission.
4. Ibid.

5. James Currie, M.D., *Medical Reports on the effects of cold and warm water as a remedy in fever and other Diseases* (London: Printed for T. Cadell and W. Davis, 1805), vol 1:1-4.
6. *History of Bathing.*
7. Ellen G. White, *The Desire of Ages* (Mountain View, Calif.: Pacific Press Publishing Association, 1898), p. 195.

Chapter 4

"Those who eat flesh are but eating grains and vegetables at second hand; for the animal receives from these things the nutrition that produces growth. The life that was in the grains and vegetables passes into the eater. We receive it by eating the flesh of the animal. How much better to get it direct, by eating the food that God provided for our use!"— Ellen G. White, *The Ministry of Healing*, p 313.

Nutrition

This section will discuss:

- The anatomy of the gastrointestinal tract.
- The diet given to man at creation.
- The Flood and introduction of animal flesh in the diet.
- Change in longevity after the Flood.
- The vegetarian diet—Is it adequate?
- Obesity—a result of overeating and lack of exercise.
- Cholesterol and fats.
- Nuts as protective foods.
- Vegetarianism and cancer.
- Milk and milk products and eggs.

Prescription No. 3:

Nutrition

■ Cut out all animal products, including milk, milk products, and eggs. Use soy drinks and other soy products as milk and meat substitutes.

■ Try two meals a day: Start the day with a big breakfast of cooked oatmeal with dried fruits and nuts (such as a few almonds, pecans, walnuts, and ground flax seeds), a banana, and a glass of soymilk. The second meal should be eaten around 4 p.m. If you need something before going to bed, eat a piece of fruit, or preferably, drink a glass of water.

■ Eat plenty and a variety of vegetables, beans, and fruits. (Vegetarian recipes are available.) Use only whole-grain breads and cereals. Drastically reduce or, preferably, totally eliminate all refined sugars.

After fresh air and water, the third Natural Remedy is based on the concept that we need proper and adequate nutrition in order to be healthy and to stay that way.

Nutrition is a broad and complex subject. It is impossible to cover all of its aspects in one chapter, and frankly, this is truly not my aim. My purpose is not so much to give scientific facts as to point to basic, simple, natural principles of nutrition and to document that they are as old as our earth—for they were given by God at creation, as pointed out in the Bible.

It's been said, "We are what we eat." This is because the food we eat is broken down through digestion and then absorbed from the intestinal tract into the bloodstream, from which its nutrients reach and nourish every cell in the body.

So for good nourishment of our bodies, we need also, in addition to using proper food, to have properly functioning digestive, circulatory, and respiratory systems. Oxygen, from the respiratory system, combines with the nutrients from our foods to give us energy.

Digestion begins in the mouth. It is enhanced by adequate chewing, grinding, and mixing with saliva, mucus, and an enzyme, ptyalin (salivary amylase). The food in the mouth is on its way to chemical reactions. The smaller the particles, the quicker and more efficient will be the chemical reactions. The properly chewed food mass is swallowed and then propelled along the esophagus all the way to the anus, through peristaltic waves produced by the contraction of muscles within the wall of the gastrointestinal tract.

Of course, for contraction of muscles, the nervous system is also involved and must also function adequately.

Each segment of the gastrointestinal tract has its specific function.

The stomach, which receives the food from the esophagus, continues digestion to a great extent by acting as an agitator, thoroughly mixing the food with gastric juices, which contain hydrochloric acid, intrinsic factor, mucus, and enzymes.

The passage of the food into the small bowel is regulated by a muscular sphincter—the pylorus—at the end of the stomach. This regulation is important for the completion of digestion within the much smaller caliber duodenum, which receives—in addition to its own secretions—bile from the liver, and pancreatic enzymes. Bile breaks down fats. The pancreas, in addition to enzymes that break down proteins and fats, also secretes insulin for the metabolism of sugar in the bloodstream—its endocrine function. The small bowel is divided into three parts: the duodenum, the jejunum, and the ileum. This division is arbitrary, as the three segments are not readily separable anatomically. What the small bowel lacks in width is made up for in length. It is twenty-two feet long (range fifteen to thirty feet) in the average individual. Absorption, for the most part, takes place in the small bowel.

From the terminal ileum, the food is propelled into the large bowel and rectum, where mostly water, electrolytes, and in much reduced amounts, the final products of digestion are absorbed. The large bowel and rectum also provide temporary storage for waste products, which serve as a medium for bacterial synthesis of some vitamins.

The complexity of the process of digestion alone, with the multiplicity of chemical reactions which must take place in an orderly fashion, makes one exclaim, as did David in Psalms 139:14: "I will praise thee; for I am fearfully and wonderfully made: marvelous are thy works, and that my soul knoweth right well!"

Our omniscient God, who made our bodies, with all their complexities—the digestive system being just one of those—gave us at creation the diet which best nourishes us. It is comparable to car manufacturers giving us a manual for the proper care of the automobile we purchase from them.

Genesis 1:29 says: "And God said, behold I have given you every herb bearing seed, which is upon the face of all the earth, and every tree in the which is the fruit of a tree yielding seed; to you it shall be for meat." Grains, fruits, and nuts were given at creation. What about vegetables? They were added after Adam and Eve disobeyed. And interestingly, they were added as part of the curse that their sin brought on them and on Planet Earth. Genesis 3:18: "Thorns also and thistles shall it [the ground] bring forth to thee; and thou shalt eat the herb of the field."

It seems that a change occurred in the human body after the entrance of sin, which made the eating of vegetables necessary, or important. Interesting thought, isn't it? That's one of the questions I will have for God when I see Him face to face. But then, knowing the beneficial effects of green vegetables (as sources of fiber, vitamins, minerals, phytochemicals, and antioxidants), we can detect God's love and concern even in the curse!

So we accept, from a biblical basis, that the original diet God gave to man consisted of grains, fruits, nuts, and vegetables—a meat-free, cholesterol-free, fiber-rich, vegetarian diet. A diet moderate in protein content, free of refined nutrients (whether sugar, protein, or fat), and rich in complex nutrients—especially carbohydrates. A diet as "natural" as it comes from the ground. By the way, this term *natural* is a misnomer when used in any context of refinement, separation, or production of food. Once nutrients are separated from their original environment, that food item is no longer "natural." The Author of life has placed in each fruit, nut, grain, and vegetable the right elements—in proper quality and quantity—for their easy digestion and absorption by our gastrointestinal tract and for the nourishment of our bodies.

Based on the Bible, animal flesh became necessary after the Flood. Genesis, chapter 7, gives the account of the Flood. After Noah and his family entered the ark, there also came in "clean beasts by sevens, the male and his female, and unclean beasts by two, the male and his female, . . fowls also of the air by sevens, the male and female: to keep seed alive upon the face of all the earth" (Genesis 7:2, 3). "The waters prevailed exceedingly upon the earth, and all the high hills . . . and the mountains were covered" (verses 19, 20). It rained for forty days (verse 17). But the waters covered the earth for 150 days. "All flesh died, and . . . every living substance was destroyed" (verses 21, 23).

But God remembered Noah. Genesis, chapter 8, gives a beautiful account of the aftermath of the Flood with the raven and the dove, and the covenant made between God and Noah, as He instructed Noah and his family to descend from the ark and to bring forth with him all the cattle, fowl, and creeping things that had been preserved within the ark.

It is reasonable to assume that a torrential downpour of rain for forty days, the breaking up of the fountains of the deep (Genesis 7:11), and the earth being completely covered for 150 days to a depth of fifteen cubits (twenty-two and a half feet) over the highest mountain peaks—through unimaginable mudslides and avalanches—caused utter havoc to the earth's surface, destroying all edible food. So God instructed Noah, in Genesis 9:3, 4, that "every moving thing that liveth shall be meat for you: even as the green herb have I given you all things. But flesh with the life thereof, which is the blood thereof, shall ye not eat."

Thus, meat eating, of necessity, was introduced into the diet.

In *Nutrition for Vegetarians*, Drs. Agatha M. and Calvin L. Thrash state: "On man's original diet of fruit, nuts, legumes, and probably fruit and vegetables, the average recorded lifespan was 912 years (Genesis 5:3-22). Animal products were permitted in man's diet after the Flood (Genesis 9:3) . . . the average for the first ten generations after the Flood . . . was but 317 years" (Genesis 11:10-32; Genesis 25:7, 8)[1]

The steady decline continued until reaching the three score and ten (70 years of age) level by the time of the exodus of the children of Israel from Egypt 430 years later, as stated by Moses in Psalms 90: "The days of our years are threescore years and ten; and if by reason of strength they be fourscore years, yet is their strength labour and sorrow; for it is soon cut off, and we fly away" (Psalms 90:10).

We know that a "high meat diet stimulates a rapid growth, predisposing to a shorter lifespan."[2]

Is there scientific proof of the superiority of a total vegetarian diet?

First, it must be recognized that there are many types of vegetarians. But basically, they fall into three major categories: lacto-ovo-vegetarians, who exclude all animal products except milk, milk products, and eggs from their diet; lacto-vegetarians, who allow milk and milk products but no eggs in their diet; and total vegetarians, or vegans, who are strict vegetarians, allowing no animal products whatsoever in their diet.

Several years ago in the mid-1960s, Drs. Hardinge and Stare[3] conducted some landmark studies comparing the complete diets in three groups—meat-eating Americans, pure vegetarians (vegans), and lacto-ovo-vegetarians—to previously established nutritional standards with respect to a diet providing adequate amounts of the essential amino acids, and in the right proportions to build the proteins needed for life and health. The question has always been whether a total vegetarian diet can provide adequate amounts of proteins to nourish the body.

Amino acids are used by the body as building blocks to make the proteins it needs. There are twenty such amino acids. Eight, called essential, must be provided by the food we eat. The other twelve can be manufactured by our bodies.

These two researchers, comparing the mix of amino acids in each of the subjects to the mix of the known established standards—as well as to human breast milk—found that the mix of amino acids in the total vegetarian diet most closely resembled the mix in the established standards as well as in human breast milk. It can be safely assumed, explains Neil Nedley, that "The only food specifically designed to meet all the amino acid needs of a human is human breast milk."[4]

"Compared to cow's milk (3.3 g/d), and goat's milk (4.1 g/d), the protein content of human breast milk is 1.2 g/d. It's interesting that humans double their birth weight in 120 days, cows in 47 days, and goats in 19 days. . . . A human baby fed cow's milk will not, obviously, double its birth weight in 47 days instead of 120 days. This is genetically pre-determined."[5]

What happens, then, to the excess, unutilized protein? Could it possibly harm the developing infant?

Another important consideration brought out by Dr. Nedley: "Is it necessary to eat a perfect balance of amino acids at a given meal to utilize them properly?"[6] The answer is provided by the American Dietetic Association, he points out. The association stated in 1988 that "It is the position of the American Dietetic Association that vegetarian diets are healthful and nutritionally adequate when appropriately planned."[7]

On the issue of the necessity for a full complement of proteins at each meal, the association added, "It is not necessary that complementation of amino acid profiles be precise and at exactly the same meal, as the recent popular 'combined protein theory' suggested."[8]

The reality is that a total vegetarian diet that contains fruits, grains, nuts, and vegetables is fully adequate in proteins. It has been documented, and this is a very important fact, that "every single vegetable and grain evaluated has more than twice the daily recommended amount of the 8 essential amino acids our body needs."[9]

One of the best summary statements on the

adequacy of a total vegetarian diet is provided by Dr. Mark Messina, a respected nutrition scientist who worked at the National Cancer Institute's Diet and Cancer Branch, as quoted in *Proof Positive*: "When people eat several servings of grains, beans, and vegetables throughout the day, and get enough calories, it is virtually impossible to be deficient in protein."[10] And not only that, I believe, a balanced vegetarian diet provides a better quality of protein than does a meat diet.

One of the major health considerations in America is obesity. Being overweight contributes to high blood pressure, heart disease, diabetes, cancer, arthritis, gallbladder disease, and other health problems, and is a source of major complications after surgery and other medical interventions.

Overeating and lack of exercise are the two major causes of overweight. The fat content of our diet, by itself, causes problems. Without exercise, extra fats, especially cholesterol, not burned up, accumulates in the lining of our blood vessels, causing them eventually to plug up. This interrupts the flow of oxygenated blood to the area of the body supplied by these vessels, causing death of tissues—heart attacks, stroke, gangrene of the toes and feet.

Notwithstanding the occasional debate on cholesterol, the overwhelming scientific evidence points to it as a major culprit as a cause of peripheral vascular disease. It is here that the superiority of the total vegetarian diet has been demonstrated.

As far back as 1989, population studies began to show "the protective role of plant food groups such as fruits, vegetables, legumes and cereals."[11]

Historically, efforts were directed toward identifying the type and, to some extent, the amount of dietary fat necessary to reduce the risks of heart disease.

By 1999, it became "clear that although a fat-modified diet can significantly affect cardiovascular disease risks, other components in the diet, such as fiber, plant protein, and soy protein appear to confer additional protective effects that extend beyond the lipid-lowering effects of the recommended diets."[12]

Also, in search for specific food items that could favorably affect heart disease risks, nuts emerged, and proved to have distinctive fatty acid profiles. Nuts are not only "rich sources of unsaturated fats, but, they also contain several non-fat constituents such as plant protein, fiber, micronutrients, plant sterols, and phytochemicals."[13]

In 1992, Gary Frazer, and coworkers at the Center for Health Research at Loma Linda University School of Public Health, first reported on the Adventist Health Study—a prospective cohort investigation of 31,208 non-Hispanic white California Seventh-day Adventists.[14]

This landmark investigation was completed in six years. Endpoints were the incidence of myocardial infarctions or fatal coronary heart failure. Extensive dietary questionnaires were filled out by each of the participants initially, detailing their use of sixty-five food items from never consumed, to consumed more than once a day. In addition, the participants' age, sex, weight, exercise habits, use of tobacco, alcohol, coffee, meat, and history of high blood pressure, were examined. Data were reported in three categories, and results were the same in all three categories, depending on how often the participants ate nuts: 1) less than once a week; 2) one to four times a week, or, 3) five or more times a week. The incidence of fatal heart attacks decreased from 27 percent for category 2, to 55 percent for those eating nuts five or more times a week. Whole grains and fruits were also overall protective, while beef increased the risk of myocardial infarction in men but not in women. In analyzing the data, the authors postulated some mechanisms of action:

1. The fat content of nuts, mostly monounsaturated oleic acids, varying from 48 percent to 74 percent, lowers total serum cholesterol and improves lipoprotein profile.

2. Nuts, being high in dietary fiber—4 percent to 11 percent by weight—help to lower serum LDL cholesterol (the bad cholesterol).

3. Nuts have a good quality protein ratio—14 percent to 26 percent by weight. (They are low in lysine and high in arginine amino acids.)

4. Nuts are an excellent source of tocopherols, considered the highest source of Vitamin E of any natural food except sweet potatoes. (It is known that Vitamin E reduces the oxidation of LDL cholesterol, a major contributor to atherosclerosis.)

Commenting further on the benefits of the good quality protein ratio of 14 percent to 26 percent, the authors added that it is one of the lowest among high protein foods and is the opposite of that found in meat.

What is known about the properties of arginine? Arginine relaxes and dilates blood vessels by its action on the smooth muscles within their walls. Arginine inhibits platelet aggregation, monocyte adherence, smooth muscle proliferation, and chemotaxis, thus keeping the blood thin and flowing. In addition, arginine decreases total serum cholesterol.

Since 1992, two large prospective studies have confirmed these observations.[15, 16] Also, evidence corroborating the earlier results reported by Frazer and his associates was recently summarized.[17]

Nuts are rich in the minerals typically lacking in the American diet. They are good sources of manganese, copper, magnesium, phosphorus, zinc, selenium, potassium, and iron. For example, one ounce of almonds provides 8 percent of the daily need for calcium; one ounce of Brazil nuts provides 920 percent of the recommended dietary allowance of selenium[18]; peanuts are a good source of folate; and nuts are also high in fiber, as mentioned, providing 5 percent to 10 percent of the recommended daily fiber intake in a one-ounce serving.[19]

The folic acid in nuts is thought to help lower blood homocysteine, which, if high, correlates with the severity of carotid stenosis.[20]

Walnuts, in particular, are rich in linoleic acid, which can be converted in the body to omega-3 fatty acids—the fats in fish oils. By the way, "The richest source of omega-3 fatty acids, are flaxseeds,"[21] for the consideration of those who wanted to give up fish but were concerned about their supply of omega-3 fatty acids. Omega-3s help fight heart disease and improve brain function. Combined with walnuts in equal proportions, "flax-nut butter," with its higher doses of omega-3s, "helps improve symptoms of coronary artery disease, rheumatoid arthritis, psoriasis and hypertrigliceridemia."[22]

As a general rule, the proportion of saturated fat in Western diets is higher than that in Mediterranean diets. In one recent study,[23] walnuts were substituted for typical Mediterranean foods and oils, which are rich in monounsaturated fatty acids and low in saturated fats, in order to evaluate their cholesterol-lowering potentials. The results showed a further reduction of total and LDL cholesterol levels in men and women with hypercholesterolemia. It can be, then, "concluded that greater benefits might be obtained by partially substituting walnuts for traditional Western dietary fats," stated the authors.

So, in summary, nuts provide good quality fats, proteins, dietary fiber, Vitamin E, copper, magnesium, and other minerals and trace elements, which reduce serum cholesterol, keep the blood thin, and protect the wall of blood vessels—almost the opposite effect of meat and other animal products.

People who experience ill effects from the use of nuts may find the difficulty removed by eating less.

Another important benefit of a total vegetarian diet is in its ability to fight one of the most dreaded diseases in the world—cancer. Cancer is the number 2 killer in America after heart disease. One in every four deaths is from cancer, totaling over 500,000 deaths annually. Many people fear the ravages of cancer and its treatment more than death itself. With the present high incidence of, and mortality from, cancer, I cannot help but reflect on statements made over 130 years ago by Ellen G. White:

- 1868: "The liability to take disease is increased tenfold by meat eating."[24]
- 1896: "Cancers, tumors, and all inflammatory diseases are largely caused by meat eating."[25]
- 1905: "People are continually eating flesh that is filled with tuberculous and cancerous germs. Tuberculosis, cancer, and other fatal diseases are thus communicated."[26]

When these statements were made, there was no evidence from medical research of any infectious association in cancer genesis, and, in fact, there was complete denial by the medical profession that such an association existed. Virology, established as a science in the 1940s, is providing accumulating evidence that both DNA and RNA viruses participate in the initiation and the promotion of tumorigenesis in man. (A virus consists of a small package of genetic information, either in the form of DNA or RNA, wrapped up in a structural protein coat)

Examples of virus-induced cancers in humans are:

- Hepatocellular carcinoma (primary liver cancer): Hepatitis B virus.
- Burkitt lymphoma: Epstein-Barr virus (EBV).
- Cancer of the cervix: herpes simplex virus type 2 (HSV-2).

The following statement from a major textbook of surgery gives relevance to those earlier ones made by Ellen G. White: "Induction of tumors by infectious agents was a long-disputed concept in the early part of this century" (our recent twentieth century). "Today, it is unequivocal that both RNA and DNA viruses induce tumors in animals from amphibians to primates. It has become accepted that this process also includes humans."[27]

Can there be contamination of viral particles from one species to another? International comparisons suggest that countries where more animal protein is eaten have more lymphomas. The strongest link was found between bovine (cow) protein and lymphoma.[28]

Other population studies have found an association between animal protein consumption and increased incidence of cancers of the breast, colon, prostate, kidney, and uterus (endometrium).[29]

Is the problem the animal protein per se, or is it the lack of certain nutrients found abundantly in a plant-based diet? The answer is probably both. When compared to vegetable protein, animal protein does increase cancer risk. In addition, nutrients, especially antioxidants found in plant products, appear to prevent cancer. A good example is soy. Dr. Mark Messina, noted soybean researcher, has listed a number of soy protein products that have cancer-fighting roles. "These include soy protein isolate, soy flour, and textured vegetable protein."[30] Furthermore, human population studies suggest that "soy has a role in preventing a variety of cancers including colon, rectum, prostate, stomach, lung, and breast. The evidence is that plant products often have a host of cancer-protective properties that may be of even more benefit than their superior type of protein."[31]

What about milk and milk products? Is it safe and beneficial to discard them from the diet?

I was beginning my junior year in medical school at Howard University College of Medicine (1965). It was my turn to give a short discourse on a medical or paramedical subject to members of First Church in Washington, D.C., where I was a member. (One of the practicing surgeons in D.C.—the late Dr. Neville Ottley—had set up a program in which junior and senior medical students practiced presenting to the church subjects of their choice.) I was impressed to look into advertising and how it impacted our health habits. My first "no brainer" conclusion was that the true purpose of advertising is to sell. I must have had the television set on while preparing my talk, because in looking for examples, my mind turned to milk. Back in 1965, we were being bombarded with advertising on milk. It dawned on me that as adults, we humans were the only mammals who continued to drink milk after severance from our mothers. And of course, even then we don't drink human milk, but milk from other species—cows and goats, for example. Could that of itself also present some problems? There were quite a few wide-eyed faces in the audience!

I'll note here that in 1974, the Federal Trade Commission issued a "proposed complaint" citing that the slogan "everybody needs milk" represented "false, misleading and deceptive advertising."[32]

What do we know today about cow's milk? It presents major health concerns to both infants and adults.

To infants: iron deficiency anemia, increased upper respiratory allergies/asthma/infections, early atherosclerosis, juvenile diabetes, acne, rheumatoid arthritis, dental decay, and infections.

To adults: coronary artery disease, cancer, allergies, and infections.

Neil Nedley points out that "most people trying to prevent or reverse coronary artery disease think that skim milk and 1 percent fat milk are good options. But a 1990 study showed that the best results in treating heart disease with lifestyle changes were obtained when milk was eliminated altogether from the diet. All levels of cow's milk—including skim and 1 percent fat—contain casein, a common milk protein, considered one of the worst to raise blood cholesterol."[33]

Infections are a major problem for both infants and adults who drink cow's milk. Our fast-paced society prefers cold milk taken directly from the refrigerator. We probably don't have time to boil our milk, as was done in years gone by, which eliminates bacterial contamination. Pasteurized milk still contains 20,000 bacteria and 10 coliforms per milliliter—or 5 million bacteria and 2,500 coliforms per glass of milk. It is not too uncommon to hear of outbreaks of food poisoning from salmonella-infected ice cream or cheese.

Exposure of livestock feed to antibiotics and hormones to prevent infections and boost growth, respectively, and to pesticides, causes other concerns. Some experts partly link exposure to antibiotics through milk and other animal products to the increasing antibiotic resistance seen in bacteria infecting our patient population.

As a surgical oncologist, reports in the medical literature implicating milk in the rising incidence of certain cancers caught my attention. For example, a state-by-state study on milk product consumption here in the United States showed a linear relationship with the incidence of breast cancer. "The more milk a State consumed, the greater the risk of breast cancer death in that state."[34] Studies overseas have shown a "dose response" incidence of prostate cancer with the number of glasses of milk drunk per day. "Men drinking 1-2 glasses of milk per day increased their risk by 20%. The risk jumped up remarkably with more than 2 glasses per day."[35] A study from Spain found that "use of milk products triples the risk of cancer of the rectum."[36]

Until recently, two rather startling statements regarding cheese, made a long time ago by Ellen G. White, had me puzzled. When I first read them several years ago, I knew of no scientific facts available for their explanation. But as has been my practice in such situations, without being able to scientifically explain it, I followed the advice and discarded cheese from my diet. In 1868, she stated: "Cheese should never be introduced into the stomach."[37] Again, in 1905: "Butter is less harmful when eaten on cold bread than when used in cooking; but as a rule, it is better to dispense with it altogether. Cheese is still more objectionable; it is wholly unfit for food."[38]

Further scientific research may provide additional reasons for such remarkable statements condemning such a universally accepted food item as cheese. But recent documented mind-altering effects have been sufficient to justify the objection to their use. "Two biogenic amines found in cheeses, as well as in wines, and other rich foods, Tyramine and Tryptamine, act as 'false neurotransmitters' that confuse the brain. The brain confusion is brought about by the release of norepinephrine as the result of stimulation of the body's stress hormone system, which, also, causes decrease blood flow to the brain."[39]

Neil Nedley explains, "Tyramine, while acting as a neurotransmitter comes from the food we eat, so, in essence, it claims to bear a message to the brain cells, but in reality there is no message. In other words, it causes mental confusion from false communication."[40]

Tryptamine is known for its mind-altering effects. It's been associated with nightmares and is classed with drugs such as LSD, because it is hallucinogenic. Most foods containing Tryptamine also have Tyramine. Examples are: cheese, fish, sausages, and early spoilage of poultry. "Tryptamine, when combined with alcohol in the presence of helicobacter pylori (common stomach dwelling bacteria) give rise to members of the Harman family—a class of chemicals with known cancer-causing properties, as well as mental effects. Harman compounds are also found in beer and wine, and some of the mind-altering effects of alcohol, as well as the cancer risks of alcohol may be related to Harmans. Harmans, it is believed, may even perpetuate the desire for alcohol."[41]

What about eggs?

The eating of no more than three eggs per week has been advised for some time, due to their high cholesterol content. Patients with elevated blood cholesterol or history of arteriosclerotic heart disease are often told to markedly reduce or altogether stop egg consumption. What is perhaps less well appreciated is that fatal cancers of both colon and ovaries have been linked to egg consumption. "A Yale University study found that for each additional 100 mg of egg cholesterol a woman averaged per day, she had a 42% increased risk of ovarian malignancy developing."[42] "Egg consumption is also positively associated with death from prostate cancer."[43]

We conclude this chapter on nutrition realizing that there is so much more that could be said. However, evidence presented here should sufficiently point to the superiority of a total vegetarian diet. Animal protein, whether from meat, milk, or eggs, has contributed to a host of degenerative diseases, the biggest being heart disease and cancer. A lot could also be said regarding animal protein's contribution to diabetes, osteoporosis, kidney failure, kidney stones, and arthritis, to name but a few.

Plant sources of nutrition are generally modest in protein and reasonable in fat content. They do not contain cholesterol and are rich in complex carbohydrates and antioxidants.

So in recommending total vegetarianism, we refer to a diet of whole (unrefined) grains, vegetables, fruits, and nuts: the diet God gave us at creation.

If we were all to adopt a total vegetarian diet, we could by doing so prevent a host of diseases, improving both the quality and quantity of our life, and making a huge difference in the health of the entire country. We would significantly decrease the cost of health care (by disease prevention), and have enough food to feed the entire planet, thus wiping out starvation. Second-hand feeding—raising cattle and poultry to feed humans—is tremendously costly and inefficient. It also involves the use of a tremendous amount of water, by the way!

The "Old Bible" is not so old after all!

Notes:

1. Agatha Moody Thrash, M.D. and Calvin L. Thrash, Jr., M.D. *Nutrition for Vegetarians* (Seale, Alabama: New Lifestyle Books, 1982) p. 2.
2. Ibid., p. 1.
3. M. G. Hardinge, H. Crooks, F.I. Stare, "Nutritional Studies of Vegetarians," *J. Am. Diet. Assoc.*, 48 (1): pp. 25-28.
4. Neil Nedley, M.D., *Proof Positive: How to Reliably Combat Disease and Achieve Optimal Health through Nutrition and Lifestyle* (Ardmore, Oklahoma: Quality Books, Inc., 1998) p. 149.
5. Ibid., p. 149.
6. Ibid.
7. Position of the American Dietetic Association: Vegetarian Diet—Technical Support Paper, *J. Am. Diet. Assoc.*, 88(3): pp. 352-355.
8. Ibid.
9. Neil Nedley, M.D., *Proof Positive*, p. 151.
10. M. Messina, V. Messina, K.D. Setchell, *The Simple Soybean and Your Health* (Garden City Park: Avery Publishing Group, 1994), p. 24.
11. National Research Council. *Diet and Health: Implications for reducing chronic disease risk*, Washington, D.C.: National Academy Press, 1989.
12. Joan Sabate, "Nut consumption, vegetarian diets, ischemic heart disease risk, and all-cause mortality: evidence from epidemiologic studies," *Am. J. Clin. Nutr.*, 1999; 70(Suppl):500S-3S
13. Penny M. Kris-Etherton, Shaomei Yu-Poth, Joan Sabate, Hope E. Ratcliffe, Guiziang Zhao, and Terry D. Etherton, "Nuts and their bioactive constituents: effects on serum lipids and other factors that affect disease risk," *Am. J. Clin. Nutr.*, 1999. 70(Suppl):504S-11S
14. Gary E. Frazer, Joan Sabate, W. Lawrence Beeson, T. Martin Strahan, "A possible protective effect of nut consumption on risk of coronary heart disease—The Adventist Health Study," *Arch. Intern. Med.*, 1992; 152:1416-1424.

15. L.H. Kushi, A.R. Folsom, R.J. Prineas, P.T. Mink, Y. Wu, R.M. Bostick, "Dietary antioxidant, Vitamins and Death from coronary heart disease in postmenopausal women," *N. Engl. J. Med.*, 1996; 332:1156-1162.

16. F.B. Hu, M.J. Stampfer, J.E. Manson, E.B. Rimm, G.A. Colditz, B.A. Rosner, et al, "Frequent nut consumption and risk of coronary heart disease in women: Prospective Cohort Study," *BMJ*, 1998; 317:1341-1345

17. "Nuts and Effects on Lipids," *Current Opinions in Lipidology*, 2001; 12:61-69.

18. National Research Council, *Recommended dietary allowances.* 10th ed. Washington, D.C.: National Academy Press, 1989.

19. *Code of Federal Regulations* Title 21. Chapter 1. 101.9 "Nutritional labeling of food," 1999

20. J. Selhub, P.F. Jacques, A.C. Bostom, et al., "Association between plasma homocysteine concentrations and extracranial carotid artery stenosis," *N. Engl. J. Med.*, 1995; 332:286-291.

21. Neil Nedley, M.D. *Proof Positive*, p. 122.

22. Ibid., pp. 122, 123.

23. Daniel Zambon, Joan Sabate, Sonia Munoz, Betina Campero, Elena Casals, Manuel Marlos, Juan Laguna, and Emilio Ros, "Substituting Walnuts for Monounsaturated Fat improves the serum lipid profile of Hypercholesterolemic men and women—A Randomized Cross over Trial," *Ann. Intern. Med.*, 2000; 132:538-546.

24. Ellen G. White, *Testimonies for The Church*, vol. 2, (Mountain View, Calif.: Pacific Press Publishing Association, 1868), p. 64.

25. Ellen G. White, *Extracts From Unpublished Testimonies*, 1896. Compiled in *Counsels on Diet and Foods* (Washington, D.C.: Review and Herald Publishing Association, 1938), p. 388.

26. Ellen G. White, *The Ministry of Healing*, (Mountain View, Calif.: Pacific Press Publishing Association, 1905), p. 313.

27. L. J. Greenfield, Editor-in-Chief, *Surgery: Scientific Principles and Practice* (Philadelphia: Lippincott-Raven), p. 463.

28. A.S. Cunningham, "Lymphomas and Animal-Protein Consumption," *Lancet*, 1976, Nov. 27; 2 (7996): 1184-1186.

29. B. Armstrong, R. Doll, "Environmental factors and cancer incidence and mortality in different countries, with special reference to dietary practices," *Int. J. Cancer.*, 1975. Apr 15; 15(4); 617-631.

30. Neil Nedley, M.D. *Proof Positive*, p. 157.

31. Ibid., p. 158.
32. *New York Times*, "Federal Trade Commission Finds Milk Advertising Campaign Deceptive," April 1974 (as quoted by Neil Nedley, M.D., in *Proof Positive*, p. 237).
33. Neil Nedley M.D. *Proof Positive*, p. 244.
34. S.P. Gaskill, W.L. McGuire, et al., "Breast Cancer Mortality and Diet in the United States," *Cancer Res.*, 1979 Sep; 39(9): 3628-3637.
35. C. La Vecchia, E. Negri, et al., "Dairy Products and the Risk of Prostatic Cancer," *Oncology*, 1991; 48(5): 406-410.
36. E. Benito, A. Obrador, et al., "A Population-based case-control Study of Colorectal Cancer in Majorca I—Dietary Factors," *Int. J. Cancer*, 1990, Jan 15: 45(1): 69-76.
37. Ellen G. White, *Testimonies for The Church*, vol. 2 (Mountain View, Calif.: Pacific Press Publishing Association, 1868), p. 68.
38. Ellen G. White, *The Ministry of Healing*, (Mountain View, Calif.: Pacific Press Publishing Association, 1905), p. 302.
39. Neil Nedley, M.D., *Proof Positive*, pp. 275, 276.
40. Ibid.
41. Ibid.
42. H. A. Risch, M. Jain, et al., "Dietary Fat Intake and Risk of Epithelial Ovarian Cancer," *J. Natl. Cancer Inst.*, 1994, Sep 21; 86(18): 1409-1415.
43. D.A. Snowdon, "Animal Product Consumption and Mortality because of all causes combined, Coronary Heart Disease, Stroke, Diabetes, and Cancer in Seventh-day Adventists," *Am. J. Clin. Nutr.*, 1988, Sep; 48(3 Suppl): 739-74

Chapter 5

"Action is a law of our being. Every organ of the body has its appointed work, upon the performance of which its development and strength depend. The normal action of all the organs gives strength and vigor, while the tendency of disuse is toward decay and death. . . . Exercise quickens and equalizes the circulation of the blood, but in idleness the blood does not circulate freely, and the changes in it, so necessary to life and health, do not take place."— Ellen G. White, *The Ministry of Healing*, pp. 237, 238.

Exercise

In this section we discuss:
- Gardening as physical activity.
- Types of exercise.
- Cardiovascular benefits of regular, moderate aerobic exercise.
- Risk/benefit ratio of exercise.
- Other benefits of regular, moderate aerobic exercise.
- Heart rate as best indicator of an effective exercise program.
- Importance of warm-up and cool-down periods before and after exercise, respectively.
- Importance of muscle building with aerobic exercise.
- Exercise and the aging process.

Prescription No. 4:

Exercise

After adequate stretching exercise of all major muscle groups and joints (one to two minutes each), walk briskly for thirty to forty minutes, preferably early in the morning when the air is fresh and filled with negative ions. Remember to fill your lungs by taking deep breaths as you walk along.

The fourth Natural Remedy is exercise. Let's think of it simply in terms of activity. Our bodies—with over 200 bones and joints and about 600 different muscles—were made for motion.

It is significant to me as a creationist that God, at creation, placed Adam in a garden. We read in Genesis 2:8: "And the Lord God planted a garden eastward in Eden, and there He put the man whom He had formed." And in verse 15: "And the Lord God took the man, and put him into the garden of Eden to dress it and to keep it." Cultivation of the soil, or gardening, to this day is recognized as one of the best forms of physical activity. It also does wonders for the emotions and mental and spiritual health. In her book *The Ministry of Healing*, as concerns care of the sick, Ellen G. White states: "Exercise in the open air should be prescribed as a life giving necessity. And for such exercises there is nothing better than the cultivation of the soil."[1] This statement, obviously influenced by Genesis 2:8, was made in 1905—far in advance of medical practice.

I completed my surgical training in 1971 and can recall patients remaining in bed for one to two days, and hospitalized for seven to eight days, after relatively minor operations. Today, of course, these same procedures are done on a "same-day" outpatient basis. Better surgical techniques are partly responsible for this change in hospital length of stay, but the recognition of medical practitioners for the need of quick postoperative activity has much to do with the improved recovery achieved today in health care.

Vernon Foster, M.D., points out that the pioneer work of Dr. Kenneth H. Cooper with the National Aeronautic and Space Administration (NASA) has greatly contributed to our understanding of exercise and its benefits. Both the U.S. Army and Air Force continue to use Dr. Cooper's research material in their training programs. It is felt that "the steady drop in coronary artery disease in America is probably due to decreased smoking and public consciousness of the importance of physical fitness and exercise, both profoundly impacted by Dr. Cooper."[2]

Five types of exercise are recognized by experts:

- Isometric (muscle contraction without motion).
- Isotonic (muscle contraction with motion, also called isophasic).
- Isokinetic (weight lifting against gravity, with muscle energy to return the weight to its original position).
- Anaerobic (exercise done while holding one's breath).
- Aerobic (exercise demanding oxygen), which requires rhythmic motion of large muscle groups.

These five types have been well documented—through research at the Cooper Aerobic Center in Dallas, Texas—as improving the status of the cardio-respiratory system and its ability to transport and deliver oxygen to needed body parts. It is believed that optimum fitness can be achieved and maintained by jogging or brisk walking thirty to forty minutes, four or five times a week, consistently and on a regular basis. It is preferable to exercise every other day rather than four straight days followed by resting for three days. Three days of rest allows some of the fitness to be lost. One can lose 50 percent of one's fitness in five weeks of inactivity. After ten weeks of inactivity, one will be back to square one and will have to start over again. The body's peak efficiency needs regular work and can be achieved in four to eight weeks on a regular exercise program.

News reports in recent months and years—of famous professional and young college athletes suddenly collapsing and dying of heat exhaustion and heart attacks during exercise—have left many puzzled and confused.

The risk/benefit ratios of exercise have been carefully weighed through research. It can be stated that "the benefits of exercise far outweigh the risks when moderate exercise programs are engaged in regularly by adults. However, with increasing amounts and intensity of exercise, the risks expand exponentially. In other words, brisk walking for 30-45 minutes realizes many more benefits than risks. However, an aerobic exercise program that is excessive in amount (more than 45 minutes), and intensity (very hard running or aerobic dance), escalates the risks sharply."[3]

So it is recommended to consult with one's physician before launching on a regular aerobic exercise program. "People who smoke, have high blood pressure, high blood cholesterol levels, and/or have parents or siblings who have died before age 50 from heart disease, should have a thorough checkup before starting to exercise. With physician's approval, a moderate exercise program, such as brisk walking, is safer than vigorous forms of exercise such as running."[4]

There are other benefits to a regular, moderate aerobic exercise program:

1. It helps "combat depression, and alleviates anxiety, substance abuse disorders, and attention deficit hyperactivity disorder (ADHD). It seems as good as medications for reducing depression. It does that by increasing serotonin and norepinephrine levels in the brain—which are neurotransmitters that can reduce depression."[5]

2. It improves insulin sensitivity, so diabetics who exercise are better able to control their blood glucose levels. They should be careful, however. Too low a blood glucose level can lead to coma. Insulin-dependent diabetics should definitely consult their physician to balance their insulin requirements and their exercise program.

3. It strengthens bones by increasing their mineral content. Osteoporosis in elderly women can actually be reversed with a regular exercise program.

4. It decreases risks of breast and colon cancer. That may be because food passes quickly through the intestinal track of active people.

5. It promotes a better functioning immune system, while excessive exercise, such as marathon running, may depress immune function. "In a study conducted on 2,300 Los Angeles marathon runners, Dr. David C. Nieman, of the School of Public Health, Loma Linda University, found that flu and colds were increased 600% in the runners who ran the L.A. marathon as opposed to runners who decided not to run it."[6]

6. It decreases the risk of gallstones.

7. It improves fibromyalgia.

An individual's heart rate is the best indicator of the effectiveness of his or her exercise program. Several formulas can be used to establish a target heart rate. "The formula used at the Cooper's Center is as follows:

■ For a man, 205 minus 1/2 his age; for a woman, 220 minus her age. Thus, a 40-year-old man would have a maximum heart rate of 185 (205-20)

■ A 40-year-old woman would have a target rate of 180 (220-40).

■ The next calculation is to take 65% to 80 % of the target heart rate to determine a proper aerobic activity. It is probably best to start at 65%, and work up to 80%."[7]

Exercise should be for twenty to thirty minutes, maintaining a heart rate as close to target as possible in order to maximize aerobic benefits.

Exercise should be enjoyable. Walking is the easiest, finest, cheapest activity one can do. Others, of course, are: swimming, outdoor cycling, cross-country skiing, jogging, or running.

Exercise should always begin with a warm-up. This serves to increase the body's temperature and to stretch the muscles gradually. Warm-up should last five minutes and include stretching arm and leg muscles, forward bending, back stretching, and jogging in place.

With the twenty to thirty minutes of aerobic activity in which the target heart rate is reached, some muscle-building activity should be included, such as push-ups, sit-ups, or even weight-lifting (isotonic exercise). Before stopping altogether, a cool-down period for another five minutes, during which the pace is slowed down, is extremely important.

The "fountain of youth" has forever been a pursuit of men and women everywhere. People, for the most part, do not like to grow old.

Exercise has been proven to make a significant difference in the aging process.

David C. Nieman, D.H.Sc., in his book, *The Adventist Healthstyle*, devotes an entire chapter to the "aging process." In it, he points out that "the fastest-growing minority in the United States today is the elderly—those who reach or pass the age of 65. Nearly 30 million elderly persons live in the United States, a number that is expected to climb to 64.6 million, or 21 percent of the total population, by the year 2030."

As a surgical oncologist, more and more of the patients I see today are 70 and 80 years of age. With improved techniques of anesthesia, most of these patients tolerate one operative procedure very well. However, they do not withstand complications, and by and large do not survive additional traumatic interventions. So the elderly are not refused treatment of their cancer on the basis of age. Proper pre-operative evaluation and preparation, along with peri-operative support, are a must if they are to survive.

Published in 1992, *The Adventist Healthstyle* predicted that "by the year 2000, 3.8 million elderly people will have senile dementia, especially Alzheimer's disease."

As a person ages, "normal yet irreversible changes occur in the body . . . some of the changes . . . include a decrease in ability to taste, smell, hear, and see; loss of teeth and bone mass in the jaw area; decrease in ability to digest and absorb food; reduction in muscle and bone mass throughout the body; impairment of memory, judgment, feelings, personality, and ability to speak; decrease in reaction time and ability to balance, diminished liver and kidney function; and a decrease in heart and lung tissues.

"Interestingly, many of the changes that accompany aging are of the same type that can be expected with inactivity. In fact, much of the deterioration attributed to aging can be explained by the fact that people tend to exercise less as they age: all living cells, tissues, and organs start to age when their particular activity is impaired, and the body as a whole will age faster without regular exercise."

Nieman then ends the chapter by citing two elderly Seventh-day Adventist women who have reaped the benefits of wise lifestyle choices. The story of one of these women follows:

"Dubbed, 'Grandma Whitney' by the press here and abroad, Hulda Crooks, then, at the age of 95, had climbed Mount Whitney, in California (the highest mountain in the Continental U.S. at 14,495 feet), 23 times. Mountain climbing was not something Hulda had done all of her life. After her husband, Samuel A. Crooks, M.D. died in 1950, Hulda took to the outdoors, where nature provided 'a tranquilizer for her emotions.'

"In 1962, at age 66, . . . encouraged by her friends, Hulda climbed Mount Whitney for the first time. . .

"Hulda's body fat just before her Mount Whitney climb was 25 percent, that of a college woman. Her HDL cholesterol was 53 mg./dl., giving her a total cholesterol/HDL cholesterol ratio of 4.2, presenting below average risk of heart disease. . .

"In 1987, Dentsu Inc., Japan's largest advertising firm, thought it a novel idea to have a 91-year-old woman climb with them in celebration of the 60th anniversary of the Dentsu employees' annual climb of Mount Fuji. Hulda was sent by Loma Linda's mayor Elmer Digneo as an 'ambassador of goodwill and healthful living.'

"On July 24, 1987, Hulda watched the sunrise from the top of Mount Fuji. Six weeks later she was on top of Mount Whitney once again. Hulda became the oldest woman in the history of Japan to climb Mount Fuji and the oldest person, man or woman, to climb Mount Whitney. These back-to-back achievements caught the attention of the world press, and Hulda's story was told and retold in the media from China to the United States.

"Hulda's achievements, as laboratory test have proved, are not because of unique genetic endowments. . .

"Hulda was born and raised on a Canadian farm, where she grew up on a non-vegetarian diet of meat, milk, cream, butter, eggs, and plenty of vigorous physical activity. In her father's country store, she had free access as well to a large barrel of hard candy at one end of the counter and soft-centered chocolates at the other. By age 16, at the height of only 5 feet six inches, she weighed 160 pounds despite her physical activity. At 18, '...she joined the Seventh-day Adventist Church' . . . and '...became a lacto-ovo-vegetarian. For more than 75 years she has followed this diet. . .' consisting of . . . a wide variety of fruits, vegetables, whole grains, and nuts, with moderate amount of low fat milk and a few eggs. A computerized analysis of her diet showed more than half of the nutrients coming from carbohydrates (59 percent carbohydrates, 25 percent fat), with vitamins A, C, and E at two to three times the recommended level.' and that, 'without the use of any supplements.'

"Hulda's achievements . . . are the result of proper health stewardship—lifestyle rooted in a deep faith in God and balanced by regular exercise, sufficient rest, and a vegetarian diet. The vitality of Hulda Crooks is within the reach of most people who make the same choice of lifestyle."[8]

"Dr. Paul W. White...states: '. . . the best way to keep fit is to walk and walk and walk. And that's my type of exercise."[9]

So in conclusion, moderate, aerobic exercise, entered into with caution and preparation, can be of great benefit to one's state of health, and with consistency, can contribute to one's longevity, with excellent quality.

Just like fresh air, pure water, and good nutrition, exercise—the fourth Natural Remedy—can do more for us than a handful of pills. God designed it at creation.

Notes:

1. Ellen G. White, *The Ministry of Healing*, (Mountain View, Calif.: Pacific Press Publishing Association, 1905), p. 265.
2. Vernon W. Foster, M.D., *NewStart: New Health, New Energy, New Joy!* (Santa Barbara: Woodbridge Press, 1988), p. 88.
3. Melvin Beltz, M.D., *Wellness to Fitness* (Hermosa, South Dakota: Black Hills Health and Education Center, 1991), p. 10.
4. Ibid., p. 11.
5. Neil Nedley, M.D., *Depression—The Way Out* (Ardmore, Oklahoma: Nedley Publishing, 2001), p. 81.
6. Melvin Beltz, M.D., *Wellness to Fitness*, p. 13.
7. Vernon W. Foster, M.D. *NewStart*, p. 84.
8. David C. Nieman, D.H.Sc., *The Adventist Healthstyle* (Hagerstown, Maryland: Review and Herald Publishing Association, 1992), pp. 112-122.
9. Ibid., p. 119.

Chapter 6

"Some make themselves sick by overwork. For these, rest, freedom from care, and a spare diet, are essential to restoration of health. To those who are brain weary and nervous because of continual labor and close confinement, a visit to the country, where they can live a simple, carefree life, coming in close contact with the things of nature, will be most helpful. Roaming through the fields and the woods, picking the flowers, listening to the songs of the birds, will do far more than any other agency toward their recovery."—Ellen G. White, *The Ministry of Healing*, pp. 236, 237.

Rest

In this section we discuss:
■ The rhythm of life.
■ Experience in Great Britain with a weekly day of rest.
■ The weekly cycle.
■ Work-rest principle.
■ The Sabbath rest.
■ Two types of fatigue.
■ Insomnia and melatonin.
■ Production of melatonin in the body.
■ Sleep requirements with age.

Prescription No. 5:

Rest

Be in bed by 10 p.m. every night. Every hour slept before midnight is extremely beneficial. Get eight hours of sleep every night. Remember also to take one day each week as a complete break from all stresses, for rest of body and mind.

Our previous chapter dealt with exercise. We concluded that exercise, the fourth Natural Remedy, can do more for us than a handful of pills.

Exercise, or activity, however, depletes our body's stores of energy. In order to stay healthy, these energy stores must be restored or replenished. This is accomplished by rest or relaxation. To maintain vibrant health there must be balance between activity and relaxation. The late Dr. Vernon Foster coined it, "the rhythm of life."[1]

This balance is everywhere, whether within our body mechanism, or governing the celestial bodies. God ordained it at creation. In Genesis 1:3-5, we read: "And God said, let there be light: and there was light. And God saw the light, that it was good: and God divided the light from the darkness. And God called the light day, and the darkness He called night, and the evening and the morning were the first day." And so it was said at the close of the succeeding five days of creation (Genesis 1:8, 13, 19, 23, 31).

After the Flood, God established the four seasons and made a vow to Himself that "While the earth remaineth, seedtime and harvest, and cold and heat, and summer and winter and day and night shall not cease" (Genesis 8:22).

The heart is the best example in our body of the balance between activity and rest. After every contraction, a brief rest period follows. During this resting period, the heart is nourished with oxygen and nutrients, enabling it to continue to work at peak efficiency for eighty or more years.

This cycle of work and rest exists in every organ and cell of our body. Keeping pace with, and cooperating with, that rhythm promotes good health.

We live in a society today where work, if not balanced by rest, can be "an oppressive and unrelenting master. Unrelenting work patterns can degrade human personality, destroy the equilibrium between body and spirit, and turn a person into a brute. This was true in the ancient agricultural societies where dependent workers were often oppressed and exploited by unscrupulous masters. But, it also applies to today's technological society where machines often tend to annihilate personal individuality. In some instances, it is insatiable greediness that drives people to work uninterruptedly, thus becoming slaves of greater gain."[2] "God was well aware of human vulnerability to lucrative ambitions," so He "ordained not only work, but rest also."[3]

"Rest contributes to the quality, intensity, and length of life. It also improves mental and physical efficiency."[4]

This was well proven by experience with factory workers in Great Britain during World War II:

The British government, wanting to boost production of war materials, increased the work week to seventy-four hours. Soon, however, "workers became irritable and restless. Morale dropped, accidents and spoiled work shot up."[5] The decision was immediately reversed by the government, and furthermore, the work week was further reduced to forty-eight hours. Production rose 15 percent. A law was soon passed "requiring that workers take one day of rest each week and be given at least 2 weeks of vacation each year."[6]

Says Vernon Foster, "One day of rest each week! That prescription is as old as the earth itself"[7]—and first taken by God, the Creator Himself.

In Genesis 2:1-3, we read: "Thus the heavens and the earth were finished, and all the host of them. And on the seventh day God ended His work which He had made, and He rested on the seventh day from all His work which He had made. And God blessed the seventh day, and sanctified it: because that in it He had rested from all His work which God created and made."

Why did God rest at creation?

At the beginning of this book, I pointed out that my purpose in writing was not so much to provide new scientific or medical information—which today can be easily obtained from the Internet—as to point the reader to the Creator-God and to the relevancy of His love letter, the Bible, to us.

Samuele Bacchiocchi states: "It is divine concern for human well-being which led God to ordain the pattern of six days for work and the seventh for rest."[8] God emphasized that ordination by first setting the example through His own behavior.

There is more to the seven-day weekly cycle than meets the eye. This unit of time established at creation is to me one of the most convincing evidences that the Bible is God's Word and is true.

We have nothing on earth or in the sky on which to base the origin of this unit of time. The day, the month, the year—these relate to the earth, the moon, the sun, respectively. On what do we base the seven-day weekly cycle (which, by the way, has withstood several attempts at changing it)? The only evidence of its origin is in the Bible. Except for Genesis, chapter 1, and Genesis 2:1-3, there is no other basis for a seven-day weekly cycle.

I call the seven-day week God's unit of time, which to me, He divided amazingly disproportionately: six days for man; one day for Himself. (It really should be the other way around, shouldn't it? After all, it's all His!) But it's a division for the good of man, and a prescription, following the example of the Creator.

God obviously intended to show the value of work as preceding rest. Adds Bacchiocchi: "Experience teaches us that work and rest are two genuine and significant human needs. A person who is workless is one who feels worthless. Work is needed to experience self-worth, to develop one's creative abilities, and reflect the image of the ever-active Creator. If work was needed before the fall to enhance human life with rewarding activities, how much more needed it is today when idleness lures people into all sorts of vices and crimes!"[9]

This obviously was important to God and intended to be restorative for man in the most absolute way. So important was it that God repeated it, placing it in the form of a command in the midst of the Ten Commandments, which He gave to the Israelites 3,500 years ago as they came out of Egypt.

Someone may be tempted to think that because there is no "command" to keep the Sabbath until the Israelites left Egypt, it is therefore not intended for mankind as a whole but only for the Jews. We must remember that communication at the time of the patriarchs—and until the printing page came into existence—was by word of mouth and example, which example God set Himself at creation. One is not expected to "remember" what one did not previously learn. The Israelites, having spent 400 years in Egypt, had forgotten about the Sabbath, it must be assumed. So on Mount Sinai, in the giving of the Ten Commandments, God introduces the Sabbath commandment—and only the Sabbath commandment—with "Remember."

Exodus 20:8-11 states: "Remember the Sabbath day to keep it holy. Six days shalt thou labor and do all thy work: but the seventh day is the Sabbath of the Lord thy God: in it thou shalt not do any work, thou, nor thy son, nor thy daughter, thy manservant, nor thy maidservant, nor thy cattle, nor thy stranger that is within thy gates: for in six days the Lord made heaven and earth, the sea, and all that in them is, and rested the seventh day: wherefore the Lord blessed the Sabbath day, and hallowed it."

Comments Bacchiocchi again: "The command to rest on the seventh day is preceded by the injunction, 'six days you shall labor and do all your work . . .' This means that the work of the six days is viewed as a prelude or a necessary pilgrimage to reach the 'rest' experience of the seventh day."[10]

Indeed, after six days of work, unlike the Creator, who never tires nor slumbers, we are exhausted, and we need rest. We need a complete break from all stresses: physical fatigue, as well as grief, anxiety, discontentment, remorse, and guilt. We need rest of body, mind, and spirit.

We need, however, to distinguish physical from mental fatigue.

Physical, or *hypotonic*, fatigue occurs when muscles and other body structures are tired because of too much repeated activity. This type of fatigue, obviously, is experienced by everyone who earns his living by the sweat of his brow. Symptoms indicative of hypotonic fatigue are: loss of efficiency, decreased productivity, increased liability to injuries, and slower reactivity to outside stimuli, leading to eventual exhaustion and physical collapse if the earlier symptoms are not heeded. The treatment for physical, or hypotonic, fatigue is physical rest—sleep—the onset of which is quick. The result is restful. It is here that Ecclesiastes 5:12 applies: "The sleep of a labouring man is sweet."

On the other hand, *hypertonic* fatigue comes from too much mental or emotional stress, without a balance of rest and physical activity. Symptoms of hypertonic fatigue are: irritability, anxiety, depression, sadness, muscle tenseness, weariness, sleeplessness, headaches, backaches, and other psychosomatic disorders, which may themselves also contribute to emotional and physical exhaustion. It may even present as a streak of rebellious feelings toward people who are loved and things ordinarily enjoyed. Unlike hypotonic (physical) fatigue, the treatment for hypertonic (mental) fatigue is physical activity—exercise! Paradoxically, vigorous exercise becomes rest—not ibuprofen, nor aspirin, nor acetominophen. A brisk walk for at least thirty minutes—swimming, tennis, handball, or whatever—just exercise, is what's needed! The worst thing to do is to sit down in that soft chair, watch TV, or take a pill. "In short, to lessen the effect of mind and nervous system fatigue [hypertonic fatigue], use muscular or physical activity."[11]

Apart from dealing with hypertonic and hypotonic fatigue, a major national problem is insomnia—the inability of people needing sleep to fall asleep when they go to bed.

In *Proof Positive*, Neil Nedley dedicated an entire chapter to "Melatonin: Agent for Rest and Rejuvenation." This segment on insomnia relies exclusively on that chapter.

In the United States, "3.3 million patients each year visit their doctors for insomnia."[12]

In 1993, research carried out at the Massachusetts Institute of Technology demonstrated that "small amounts of melatonin acted as a natural sleep aid."[13] Melatonin quickly became very popular, with "24 different U.S. companies marketing it by 1995, generating millions of dollars in sales."[14]

However, some caution is called for. While in England and Canada, melatonin is considered a drug and must be prescribed by a physician for a specific medical condition, in the U.S., it is a dietary supplement, and as such does not need to be reviewed by the FDA for effectiveness or safety. While this may be welcomed by "naturalists" here in the U.S., there are potential problems. "Quality nor labeled quantity are not guaranteed; possible long-term adverse effects, or undesirable side effects are not yet known; and, as in the case of all natural supplements, there are possible dangerous interactions with prescription drugs."[15]

Melatonin is a natural hormone produced in the body, as well as found in certain foods. What is more exciting is that its production within our bodies can be boosted naturally, without resorting to taking costly supplements. "The following are the steps in the production of melatonin in the body:

1. The pineal gland draws tryptophan, an amino acid, from the blood.
2. Tryptophan is converted to serotonin in the gland.
3. Serotonin is converted to melatonin through an enzyme, N.acetyl-transferase (NAT)."[16]

It is good to recognize, however, that melatonin is not stored in the body. A daily production is needed. "This daily production can be enhanced by:

1. Exposure to bright light early in the day.
2. Avoidance of light exposure at night (sleeping in complete darkness).
3. Eating foods rich in melatonin (oats, corn, rice), tryptophan (tofu, roasted pumpkin seeds, sesame seeds, almonds, black walnuts, blackeyed cowpeas), and Vitamin B6 (sweet bell peppers, artichoke hearts, sunflower seeds).
4. Avoidance of calcium deficiency.
5. Restricting food intake in general, and
6. Practicing fasting (especially in evening hours—no eating after 5:00 p.m.)"[17]

"It is, likewise, just as important to recognize that melatonin production can be reduced by cer-

tain lifestyle factors and practices:
1. Stress.
2. Caffeine (cuts melatonin production in half for six hours).
3. Alcohol (up to 41% reduction).
4. Tobacco.
5. Non-steroidal anti-inflammatory drugs.
6. Beta- and calcium- channel blockers.
7. Anti-anxiety drugs and sleep aids.
8. Vitamin B12 (3 mg a day).
9. Anti-depressants."[18]

One cannot help but be impressed, with some reflection, on how much rest, or lack of it, and consequently chronic fatigue, may be influenced by our bodies' store of melatonin, which in turn may be directly related to our lifestyle.

A significant number of our population have the habits of staying up late at night—with increased light exposure during these hours—eating late, and then drinking several cups of coffee in the morning and throughout the day in order to stay awake and function. Just from the standpoint of melatonin production, "It would be better to go to bed early to take advantage of the night time darkness, and then rise early."[19] This recent discovery of melatonin helps give the scientific rationale behind a statement made by Ellen G. White over a century ago: "Sleep is worth far more before than after midnight. Two hours' good sleep before twelve o'clock is worth more than four hours after twelve o'clock."[20]

How much sleep is necessary?

The amount of sleep needed for optimal health changes with age. Newborn and young children, due to increased brain activity, require the most sleep—up to twenty hours a day. By adulthood, six to seven hours of sleep are needed. This continues to increase slightly until age 70, after which the need for sleep declines again. Good rest and sleep can be enhanced by: avoiding eating late in the evening and doing heavy exercise late in the day; getting fifteen to twenty minutes of sunshine early in the morning; following a regular schedule of evening routine; taking a warm bath; drinking a warm, non-alcoholic, non-caffeine drink; and reading God's Word and talking to Him in prayer before going to bed.

Even in winter, sleeping in a well-ventilated room will enhance and promote sleep. Following these steps, we will, like King David, be able to say, "I will both lay me down in peace, and sleep: for thou, Lord, only makest me dwell in safety"(Psalms 4:8).

Indeed, true safety lies in heeding the invitation of Jesus: "Come unto me, all ye that labour and are heavy laden, and I will give you rest. Take my yoke upon you, and learn of me: for I am meek and lowly in heart, and ye shall find rest unto your souls. For my yoke is easy, and my burden is light" (Matthew11:28-30).

Notes:

1. Vernon W. Foster, M.D., *Newstart: New Health, New Energy, New Joy!* (Santa Barbara: Woodbridge Press, 1988), p. 46.
2. Samuele Bacchiocchi, *Divine Rest for Human Restlessness* (Berrien Springs, Michigan: Samuele Bacchiocchi, 1980), p. 92.
3. Ibid.

4. Vernon W. Foster, M.D., *Newstart*, p. 48.
5. Ibid.
6. Ibid.
7. Ibid.
8. Samuele Bacchiocchi, *Divine Rest for Human Restlessness*, p. 91.
9. Ibid., pp. 91, 92.
10. Ibid., p. 91.
11. Vernon W. Foster, M.D., *Newstart*, p. 50.
12. Neil Nedley, M.D. *Proof Positive: How to Reliably Combat Disease and Achieve Optimal Health through Nutrition and Lifestyle* (Ardmore, Oklahoma: Quality Books, Inc., 1998), p. 193.
13. A.B. Dollins, I.V. Zhdanova, et al., *Proc. Natl. Acad. Sci. USA*, 1994 Mar 1; 91(5): 1824-1828, as quoted in Neil Nedley, M.D., *Proof Positive*, p. 193.
14. Neil Nedley, M.D. *Proof Positive*, p. 194.
15. Ibid., pp. 198, 199.
16. Ibid., p. 201.
17. Ibid., p. 205.
18. Ibid., p. 206.
19. Ibid., p. 203.
20. Ellen G. White Manuscript Releases, vol. 7, p. 224. Found in: Ellen G. White Estate, *The Complete Published Ellen G. White Writings*, version 3.0 (CD-ROM), 1990, as quoted by Neil Nedley, M.D., *Proof Positive*, p. 203.

Chapter 7

"In the building of houses it is especially important to secure thorough ventilation and plenty of sunlight. Let there be a current of air and an abundance of light in every room in the house. Sleeping rooms should be so arranged as to have a free circulation of air day and night. No room is fit to be occupied as a sleeping room unless it can be thrown open daily to the air and sunshine."—Ellen G. White, *The Ministry of Healing*, pp. 274, 275.

Sunshine

In this section we will discuss:
- A creationist's viewpoint.
- The sun—its purpose and benefits.
- Health benefits derived from sunshine:
  - Production of melatonin
  - Production of Vitamin D
  - Regulation of earth temperature
  - Counteraction of Seasonal Affective Disorders (SAD)
- How much sunshine do we need?
- Etiology of skin cancer.
- The three major types of skin cancer.

Prescription No. 6:

Sunshine

Get out in the sunshine for fifteen to twenty minutes between 8:00 and 10:00 a.m., and again between 3:00 and 4:00 p.m. every day possible. Sunshine is healing. It is antiseptic. It is an anti-depressant and good for eyesight. It provides Vitamin D from the skin. Just avoid sunburn.

At the beginning of the preceding chapter, we saw how God established the "rhythm of life" at creation by dividing each twenty-four-hour cycle into day and night. In Genesis 1:14-17, we read that on the fourth day of creation, "God said, let there be lights in the firmament of the heaven to divide the day from the night, and let them be for signs, and for seasons, and for days, and years. And let them be for lights in the firmament of the heavens to give light upon the earth and it was so. And God made two great lights: the greater light to rule the day, and the lesser light to rule the night: He made the stars also. And God set them in the firmament of the heavens to give light upon the earth."

Of course, the two great lights are the sun and the moon in our solar system. Of note, they were created as soon as the earth had brought forth grass, herb yielding seed, and fruit trees, on the third day of creation (Genesis 1:11-13). All of this was done before God created animal life on the fifth and sixth days of creation. The main fuel of animal life, of course, is carbohydrate, which is manufactured by plants through the action of sunlight—photosynthesis. All animal food—whether protein, fat, or vitamins as well—is derived from sunlight. This shows thought, purpose, and planning on the part of the Creator, which cannot be denied as we read Genesis, chapter 1.

"The sun, 1.3 million times bigger than the earth, is 93 million miles away. The sun provides us with 4.69 million horsepower of energy per square mile. This energy takes only 8 minutes to travel the 93 million miles to reach us. And our earth intercepts only about 1 part in 2 billion of the energy radiating from the sun."[1]

The sun energy that reaches the earth is the right amount to keep us warm and give us the light we need. This energy reaches us in the form of electromagnetic radiation. Simply put, this electromagnetic radiation can be divided into three major classes:

- Short, invisible rays.
- Visible light, with all its colors.
- Long, invisible waves.

The short, invisible rays include cosmic, gamma, x-ray, and ultraviolet light (UV)—C, B, A. The long, invisible waves are: infrared, radio waves, and electric waves.

The atmosphere filters out much of this solar energy, allowing only one part in two billion of the sun's radiation to reach us, as we have just noted. The principal types that reach the earth's surface are the ultraviolet rays, the visible light spectrum, and the infrared rays.

"The middle of these frequencies is perceived as ordinary light, but they are actually a blend of all the colors of the rainbow—red, orange, green, blue, violet, and the various shades in-between. Sunlight helps us to appreciate . . . the beauty of a sunset, the rainbows, and the magnificent northern lights."[2] I can't help but reflect on Genesis 1:18 (last part): "And God saw that it was good."

What are some of the health benefits of sunshine?

- In the previous chapter, we saw that exposure to early morning sunshine helps the body to produce melatonin for a more restful sleep at night.

- Sunshine, as a mood elevator, helps fight depression. In northern climates, especially during the shorter days of winter, many people suffer from an entity called *seasonal affective disorder* or "SAD." Researchers in the field report lack of energy, depression, sleep disorders, and other symptoms caused by "sunlessness," which is relieved by exposure to artificial light of a specified brightness or by the arrival of spring.

- Sunshine is antiseptic. "Niels Finson won the Nobel Prize in 1903 for using sunlight to treat patients with tuberculosis . . . In the 1920s and 1930s many cures were reported in otherwise hopeless cases of extrapulmonary tuberculosis, particularly involving bones, with the use of sunlight (heliotherapy). As a result, many hospitals installed ultraviolet lamps in their operating rooms, and the corridors of tuberculosis wards. Windows facing the sun were incorporated into patients' rooms and even into operating theaters."[3] With the advent of antibiotics and modern technology, this natural remedy has been set aside. However, now, we are faced with increasing numbers of drug-resistant bacteria. It is true, today, in most of our cities, smoke and smog filter out much of the ultraviolet light from the sun. In addition, "most window glass in modern construction will filter at least 95% of the ultraviolet rays."[4] But would it not be wise that we, as healing professionals and hospital administrators, faced with the mounting numbers of in-hospital, antibiotic-resistant infections, reconsider heliotherapy through "direct or artificial sunlight or ultraviolet light, to disinfect rooms in nurseries, med-surg units, surgical and medical intensive care units?"[5]

■ Sunlight helps keep the skin healthy. Lately, because of the rise in the incidence of skin cancer, which is attributed to exposure to sunlight, we have come to think of sunlight as an enemy. Sunlight has gotten a "bad rap," to use a common expression. Its benefits far outweigh its disadvantages. Judicious exposure to sunlight toughens the skin, making it more resistant to disease itself. "Diaper rash, commonly caused by yeast organisms, can be virtually cured with sunlight exposure. Athlete's foot and even chronic psoriasis can respond."[6]

■ There is no doubt that the effect of sunshine on the skin, rather than capsules, pills, or dairy products, is the best source of vitamin

D. Exposure to sunlight warms the skin, bringing out the natural oils from the sebaceous glands in the hair follicles. Under the influence of ultraviolet light, the cholesterol contained in these natural oils under the skin is changed to vitamin D. This uses some of the body's pool of cholesterol, with the net effect of lowering total blood cholesterol. Vitamin D, the "sunshine" vitamin, helps transport calcium to bones, preventing rickets (bone deformities) in children, and osteomalacia in adults.

■ Sunshine regulates temperature, humidity, and wind circulation on earth through infrared radiation from the sun. Without infrared heat waves, our earth would be cold like the moon—uninhabitable, barren, and lifeless.

■ Sunshine stimulates the immune system—the primary defense system of the body. Very simply stated, it is mediated on the cellular level or through antibody production, either by "T" or "B" cells, respectively—the two main types of lymphocytes in the blood. The destruction of viruses, chemical toxins, and cancer cells is by "T" cells (cellular-mediated). "B" cells produce antibodies which coat bacteria and mark them for destruction. Sunshine helps increase the oxygen-carrying capacity of red blood cells. Oxygen destroys germs. Sunshine makes the neutrophils—specialized white blood cells that destroy and eliminate foreign invaders—more efficient at digesting germs. It increases the number of lymphocytes—both "T" and "B"—in the circulation, and helps a special natural killer (NK) cell in its protective role.

■ Sunshine lowers blood pressure, as it reduces blood cholesterol. Studies have documented a reduction in resting heart rate and respiratory rate as well. There is improved oxygen utilization, endurance, and muscle strength with regular exposure to sunshine.

■ Sunshine stabilizes blood sugar, through increasing the enzyme *phosphorylase*. This can last several hours following exposure to sunshine. Sunshine also stimulates the beta cells of the pancreas to a more efficient production of insulin. Just like exercise, sunshine lowers blood sugar in diabetics and tends to normalize blood sugar in hypoglycemics. So diet, plus exercise, plus sunshine, is a good formula for controlling adult-onset, type II diabetes.

Nine benefits, at least, of sunshine! I am sure there are more.

How much sunshine do we need? A general guideline for caucasian Americans is an average of fifteen to twenty minutes each day, during the mid-morning and mid-afternoon hours. Darker-skinned individuals need thirty minutes to three hours daily. We need to realize that our bodies store vitamin D, which can be used during the cold, sunless winter months. It is also important to remember that 95 percent of ultraviolet light does not pass through glass. So one must be in the sunshine to receive the full benefits of the sun.

Just don't be a sun worshiper—don't just lie there and get "roasted." This is harmful!

A few words about skin cancer:

By the time most young people get to be 18 years of age, they have received 50 percent to 80 percent of their lifetime sun exposure. If they have gotten two or three bad sunburns by then, the possibility of skin cancer developing, including malignant melanoma, is significantly increased. Two things must be present before cancer develops: an initiating factor, and a promoting factor. Viruses play a role as initiators in many cancers, and this may be the case for skin cancer. We do know that the primary promoter (carcinogen) in skin cancer is sunshine (ultraviolet light). But sunshine promotes skin cancer after sunburns. This happens when the polyunsaturated fats and the cholesterol under the skin are oxidized. Thus, the incidence of skin cancer can be reduced by avoiding sunburn (even mild sunburn), lowering body fat, increasing the fiber content of the diet, and by the use of antioxidants such as beta-carotene, vitamin A, vitamin C, and selenium.

There are three main types of skin cancer: basal cell carcinoma, squamous cell carcinoma, and malignant melanoma. Basal cell and squamous cell carcinomas are directly related to sun exposure and occur mainly in areas of the body that have been damaged by the sun—the face, the back, or the backs of the hands. The relationship of malignant melanoma to sunshine is an indirect one in that the incidence of malignant melanoma increases as one gets close to the equator, such as in the southern areas of the United States of America or the northern parts of Australia. Whereas basal cell and squamous cell carcinomas seldom metastasize, malignant melanoma, unless diagnosed very early, can metastasize and kill its victim. Malignant melanoma most often grows in a black mole that has been present for months or years, or even since birth (congenital nevus), and which characteristically begins to change size, color, texture—or which itches or bleeds. Occasionally, malignant melanoma will present "de novo." as a totally new lesion (with no preexisting mole). The characteristic signs of malignancy are obvious, and the lesion must be immediately biopsied for confirmation of the diagnosis.

Most people with malignant melanoma are fair-skinned, blue-eyed, and blonde, with ten to 100 moles on their bodies. Moles should be watched for change and biopsied if any change occurs. Again, most people with malignant melanoma, as with the other two skin cancers, have experienced sunburns two or three times as youngsters.

In closing, ancient cultures, recognizing the healing properties of sunshine, actually worshiped the sun as their god. In so doing, they worshiped the creation. God made the sun. The Bible tells us: "Worship God who made heaven and earth" (Revelation 14:7). As creator, God is able to do for us abundantly more than the sun can do. In fact, Psalms 84:11 reads: "For the Lord God is a Sun and Shield: the Lord will give grace and glory: no good thing will He withhold from them that walk uprightly." And in Malachi 4:2, we read: "But unto you that fear my name shall the Sun of Righteousness arise with healing in His wings."

Commenting on Christ as the "Sun of Righteousness," Ellen G. White states: "As a flower turns to the sun, that the bright rays may touch it with tints of beauty, so will the soul turn to the Sun of Righteousness, that heaven's light may beautify the character with the graces of the character of Christ."[7] And, "having gained . . . strength by communion with God, we may go on our way rejoicing, praising Him for the privilege of bringing the sunshine of Christ's love into the lives of those we meet."[8]

Notes:

1. *Encyclopedia Brittannica*, article, "Sunlight."
2. Melvin Beltz, M.D., *Wellness to Fitness*, (Hermosa, South Dakota: Black Hills Health and Education Center, 1991), p. 69.
3. Ibid., p. 71.
4. Ibid.
5. Ibid.
6. Ibid., p. 70.
7. Ellen G. White, *The Desire of Ages* (Mountain View, Calif.: Pacific Press Publishing Association, 1898), p. 468.
8. Ellen G. White, *In Heavenly Places* (Hagerstown, Maryland: Review and Herald Publishing Association, 1967), p. 62.

Chapter 8

"One of the most deplorable effects of the original apostasy was the loss of man's power of self-control. Only as this power is regained can there be real progress."—Ellen G. White, *The Ministry of Healing*, p. 129.

"Everyone who runs in the Olympics gives it all he has, but only one person wins the laurel wreath. That's how you should run the gospel race, giving it everything you've got. But in the gospel race, everyone who runs faithfully and finishes is a winner. Now those who compete in these games train their bodies and abstain from anything that would be harmful. They do it to win that laurel wreath which will soon fade and die, while the prize we receive is the crown of eternal life which will last forever. I don't run the gospel race aimlessly as if I don't know where the finish line is. I don't fight by boxing at shadows; I try to make every punch count. It's my own body that I hit to keep it under control, so that after preaching to others, I myself won't be disqualified" (1 Corinthians 9:24-27, *The Clear Word: An Expanded Paraphrase*, by Jack J. Blanco).

Abstemiousness, or Self-control
In this section we will discuss:
■ The meaning of temperance.
■ The socially accepted addictions:
    ■ Nicotine

- ■ Alcohol
- ■ Caffeine
■ What is "addiction," and what are the chances of recovery?
■ Overweight: result of overeating and lack of exercise.
■ The frontal lobe of the human brain and its function.
■ Lifestyle changes affecting frontal lobe function.
■ Hypnotism and its effect on the frontal lobe.
■ Hypnotic-like effects of:
  - ■ Some television programming
  - ■ Certain types of music
  - ■ Eastern type meditation—Yoga

Prescription No. 7:

Abstemiousness, or Self-control

Avoid all alcoholic beverages, coffee, and other caffeine-containing products. Avoid cigarette smoking, tobacco in all its forms, and the use of street drugs. Avoid gluttony—even of good and wholesome foods. Determine that you will keep from premarital and/or extramarital sex.

To be abstemious is to be temperate. Webster's *New World Dictionary*, college edition, defines temperance as "the state or quality of being temperate; self-restraint in conduct, expression, indulgence of appetites, etc.; moderation, originally as one of four cardinal virtues; moderation in eating and drinking, especially in drinking alcoholic liquors; total abstinence from alcoholic liquors."

Another definition states: "Temperance is complete abstinence from that which is harmful, and moderate use of that which is good."

Someone has said: "Imagine temperance as a stoplight, the red light equaling abstinence, the yellow light representing moderation, and the green light equaling appropriateness. As you go about your daily life you encounter crossroads, issues that need a decision. Practicing temperance is when you apply the imaginary stoplight to your experience."[1] For example:

1. **Exercise**. Should you, or should you not? Exercise helps you feel better, think clearer, and have more energy. Exercise improves your health. Exercise is a green light.

2. **Alcohol**. Government research reveals that "alcohol causes more than 100,000 deaths per year in the U.S. Thus, among drugs, alcohol is second only to tobacco as a cause of premature deaths in our nation, and is the third leading actual cause of death overall."[2] Alcohol also weakens our immune system. Alcohol is deadly. Alcohol is a red light.

3. **Sunshine**. It's a great germ fighter. It is wise to get fifteen to twenty minutes of sunshine

each day for adequate Vitamin D production. Sunlight is necessary for eyesight, plus it aids in relief of depression, as pointed out in the previous chapter. With its many positive factors, if abused, sunshine can cause harm. Too much exposure causes sunburns, and skin cancer. Sunshine is a yellow light. Proceed with caution!

Temperance applies to everything in life. It's self-control, not just in handling that which is harmful, but also that which is good. Remember the old saying, "Too much of a good thing can be bad for you."

Two statements, made years ago by Ellen G. White, are worth quoting here: "If our physical habits are not right, our mental and moral powers cannot be strong; for great sympathy exists between the physical and the moral."[3] And, "Recklessness in physical habits tends to recklessness in morals."[4] As human beings, we are not compartmentalized. Our physical, mental, social, and spiritual dimensions are interrelated, interdependent. One affects the other.

When one thinks of recklessness and deterioration in morals, whether on a personal or societal level, drug addiction comes to the forefront.

Surprisingly, however, we are not talking about addiction to cocaine and other "street" drugs, as damaging as this is to our society. Our discussion focuses on three socially, relatively acceptable drugs and chemicals, namely, nicotine, alcohol, and caffeine and caffeine-like substances—three addictions affecting billions the world over.

In the U.S. alone, cigarette smoking is responsible for over 400,000 premature deaths annually. To compare, alcohol is responsible for about 150,000 premature deaths, and cocaine, for about 200 to 300 premature deaths annually. One might be tempted to say, why all the fuss over cocaine?

Nicotine

In chapter 2, I pointed out that cigarette smoke contains over 4,000 toxic chemicals, including forty-three known carcinogens (cancer-causing agents). Cigarette smoking remains "public enemy number 1," as coined by the first Surgeon General's report in 1964. These carcinogens are not responsible for causing the addiction to tobacco. "Nicotine is the addictive ingredient in tobacco, and it is absorbed into the bloodstream and reaches the brain just as quickly, in a matter of seconds, whether from the lungs, during smoking, or the mouth, during chewing, or the nasal passages, during snuffing, tobacco."[5]

Nicotine is a potent psychoactive drug, and "like other drugs, i.e., heroin, alcohol, cocaine, etc., its continued use produces a highly controlled addictive pattern of behavior by activating nicotinic receptors in the central nervous system which in turn activate, among others, the dopaminergic reward system located in the mesolimbic area of the brain. This system has been shown to also mediate the addictiveness of other drugs like cocaine. This is not entirely new or recently acquired scientific knowledge. Between 1980 and 1994, every scientific panel and organization with expertise in addiction has reviewed the scientific research and has concluded that nicotine is addictive and has dependence-producing properties. . . . These organizations include, but are not limited to, the American Psychiatric Association, the World Health Organization, the American Medical Association, the American Psychological Association, the American Society for Addiction Medicine, the Royal Society of Canada, and the Medical Research Council of the United Kingdom, among others. In addition, recently released documents from within the Tobacco industry have revealed that the Tobacco industry recognized the addictiveness of nicotine as far back as 1963 and researched the effects of nicotine on the smokers' brain to understand nicotine biological effects."[6]

It is difficult to conceive of the apparent total lack of concern for human lives on the part of the tobacco industry. Forced by law to discontinue television and radio advertising, focused popular journals have been used, and billboards have been printed and targeted toward young people and poorer neighborhoods especially, where the ravages of cancer, high blood pressure, emphysema, asthma, etc., are already acutely felt.

This should cause all concerned citizens in the country and the world to rally and fight back to counteract the effect of tobacco advertising.

The example of Tobacco Free Partners (TFP), in Grand Rapids, Michigan, is to be emulated in every community. Under the leadership of Tom Peterson, M.D., medical institutions, pharmaceutical companies, the news media, county health departments, local chapters of the American Lung Association, the American Heart Association, and the American Cancer Society—together with third party payers and others—have, since July 2000, united in a collaborative effort to impact the health of the citizens in west Michigan.

With a clear mission statement—"To improve the health of communities by promoting a tobacco free future"—an all-front, four-pronged initiative has been launched, directed to:

1. Preventing the start of tobacco use (especially by children and young people).
2. Significantly reducing tobacco use.
3. Coordinating the efficiency and efficacy of tobacco control efforts in the region, and
4. Being an advocate to promote policy and system changes that affect tobacco control initiatives in the workplace, and elsewhere.

To practically attempt to reduce tobacco use, year around, community-wide "Tobacco Free for Good" classes are offered. The intervention of health care providers and administrators is being enlisted to provide a totally smoke-free environment on the campuses of all major health care institutions.

It will take this kind of systematic approach in all communities to counteract the powerful influence of tobacco advertising and to impact tobacco use in our country and our world. But this we must do! Our health and that of our children and succeeding generations depend on it!

One of the newest partners to join TFP is the oldest smoking cessation program in existence, both here in the U.S. and abroad—the Seventh-day Adventist Church "Breathe-Free Plan" to stop smoking. It was developed in the 1950s by a physician, J. Wayne McFarland, M.D., and a church pastor, Elman Folkenberg, as the "Five Day Plan to Stop Smoking," and was revised in 1985 as the "Breathe-Free Plan."

Cigarette smoking, ever discouraged by the Seventh-day Adventist Church, has always been considered both a habit and an addiction. So the plan incorporated from its beginning a combined approach to smoking cessation, with involvement of psychology, exercise, nutrition, and last but not least, recognition that *God is the agent of lasting behavior modification in human lives.* His help should be sought early, and He will not disappoint those who seek to find the strength that only He can provide. These principles, embodied in the "Breathe-Free Plan," account for its long-term success. The plan has helped twenty million people world-wide, thus far, to quit. Its proven technique provides:

- Insurance against failure.
- Ten weapons to kill an urge to smoke.
- Help for managing stress.
- Secrets to weight control without cigarettes.
- No medications to buy.
- No use of hypnotism.
- Personal guidance and support, and
- Three natural ways to prepare one's body to stop smoking.

Before leaving the topic of nicotine, one question might be asked? What prompted the Seventh-day Adventist Church to promote nonsmoking and to develop a stop-smoking program so early, in the 1950s? The following statement, first printed in 1905, was written by Ellen G. White: "Tobacco is a slow, insidious, but most malignant poison. In whatever form it is used, it tells upon the constitution; it is all the more dangerous because its effects are slow and at first hardly perceptible. It excites and then paralyzes the nerves. It weakens and clouds the brain. Often it affects the nerves in a more powerful manner than does intoxicating drink. It is more subtle, and its effects are difficult to eradicate from the system. . .

"The use of tobacco is inconvenient, expensive, uncleanly, defiling the user, and offensive to others. Its devotees are encountered everywhere. . . . Though men persist in using these poisons themselves, what right have they to defile the air that others must breathe?

"Among children and youth the use of tobacco is working untold harm. The unhealthful practices of past generations affect the children and youth today. . . . Boys begin the use of tobacco at a very early age. The habit thus formed when body and mind are especially susceptible to its effects, undermines the physical strength, dwarfs the body, stupefies the mind, and corrupts the morals."[7]

Were she writing today, she certainly would have included "girls" in that last paragraph.

In the light of what we know today, what remarkable statements these were, made in 1905 by someone with less than a third-grade education!

Indeed, one may ask, after such remarks, what took the Seventh-day Adventist Church forty years to come up with a plan to help smokers quit?

Alcohol

Let's turn our attention now to alcohol. We live in an age of drug-dependency, while claiming our independence! We wake up in the morning with a cup of coffee, we smoke, chew, or snuff tobacco throughout the day, and we end the day with a nightcap. Drugs—prescription and nonprescription—are often used for minor ills and pain, which could easily be treated by a change in our lifestyle. We rely on drugs to deal with problems, to give us more energy, to calm our nerves, and to forget our unhappy feelings.

We need to remember that all drugs have side effects. The risk-to-benefit ratio should always be considered, even with the use of legal/prescription drugs. Substance abuse can occur easily. It destroys the body.

Now, some general comments on alcoholism: Someone said, "Ever since Noah left the ark and got drunk, mankind has had problems with alcohol!"

Alcoholism affects virtually all organs of the body, with the worst effects on the brain, the liver, and the pancreas. Alcohol alters judgment, impairs self-control, stunts emotional growth, and breaks interpersonal relationships. The frontal lobe, where the will resides and where character is developed, is greatly affected, and consequently, all kinds of problems develop with alcohol abuse. Harsh words are spoken, fights ensue, lives are ruined, homes are broken. Accidents, injuries, and tragic deaths of innocent victims all result from the use of alcohol, as well as other drugs.

Alcohol is a source of concentrated calories (seven calories per gram). These calories are empty calories, lacking vital nutrients (vitamins, protein, fat, carbohydrate). Alcohol, therefore, contributes to obesity. "Mixed drinks and malt liquor contains sugar, but this is of little benefit except for converting it into fat and producing the proverbial 'beer belly.' Sugar actually tends to compound the toxic effect of alcohol."[8] "Triglycerides are increased in the blood stream causing cirrhosis of the liver."[9] And with alcoholic cirrhosis come "protein malnutrition, and a host of related diseases, including multiple Vitamin deficiencies, namely, Beriberi (lack of Vitamin B[1]), Scurvy (lack of Vitamin C), Pellagra (niacin deficiency), pneumonia, other infections"[10] and development of hepatoma (primary cancer of the liver) often associated in this country with hepatitis viral infestations.

"Alcohol causes pancreatitis, or inflammation of the pancreas."[11] This tends to heal, only to recur with severe abdominal distress, usually requiring hospitalization. If bleeding occurs from the pancreas, death is the outcome. Scarring, secondary to recurrent pancreatitis, will decrease insulin production and cause diabetes mellitus.

"Alcohol plays a very important role in the high rate of hypertension in our nation. Estimates are that up to 30 percent of all high blood pressure in American men can be related to alcohol consumption."[12] Often, they are treated with blood pressure medication, when what is needed is for the patients to stop drinking, and the blood pressure would return to normal. Says Neil Nedley: "It simply does not make sense to be taking blood pressure medicine and drinking alcohol even in small amounts."[13]

Combined with cigarette smoking, alcohol increases the risk of cancer of the mouth, the pharynx, and the esophagus. There is evidence that alcohol by itself influences the incidence of cancer of the breast, the liver, and the rectum.

Someone said: "Chronic alcoholism produces a medical [library] of diseases because of its toxicity to virtually all body tissues."

Now, specifically on alcoholic addiction: Alcohol, like nicotine, is a psychoactive drug and causes chemical dependence. This chemical dependence may begin with the very first exposure, or gradually develop over time of use. Once a person becomes a user for a period of time, there is an addiction.

Caffeine

In chapter 3, we showed how essential to life water is, both inside the body and used on the outside. More people are being made aware that our bodies need six to eight glasses of water every day to stay healthy. Though to a much lesser extent nowadays, it is not unusual, however, to find some people who haven't drunk water in years. They say they just can't, or don't like to, drink water. These people, unfortunately, substitute drinks that not only can't do what water does for the body, but that actually interfere with normal body functions and/or introduce harmful substances into the body. One of these drinks is coffee, the most popular "wake-up" drink the world over. How daring to say anything against such a popular custom—the morning cup of coffee!

But dare we must.

Coffee, and the colas, contain caffeine, which is a methylxanthine. Although their structure and biologic functions differ significantly from caffeine, other drugs of the xanthine family are theophylline, found in black tea, and theobromine, found in chocolate. The methylxanthines were found in some laboratory studies, albeit in high doses, to be "capable of damaging chromosomes of both plants and animals."[14]

In a fairly recent exhaustive review, tea—whether black, green, or oolong—was noted to be a rich source of biologically active ingredients (such as flavonoids, vitamins, and fluoride) Flavonoids, as antioxidants, neutralize the free radicals capable of causing cellular damage.[15]

However, caffeine affects the brain's communication system. Between two brain cells is a gap which contains chemical messengers, or neurotransmitters. A nerve impulse, or message, traveling through one nerve cell passes through the gap and neurotransmitter to reach its neighboring nerve cell. And of course, the neurotransmitter has the ability to interfere with the transmission of that nerve impulse—stimulating, or depressing, or, blocking, it altogether. General anesthesia, for example, is a controlled way of blocking the nerve impulse altogether, allowing us to be put to sleep for an operation and to be awakened at the end of the procedure.

Two important neurotransmitters are affected by caffeine. They are acetylcholine and adenosine. Acetylcholine stimulates nerve transmission, while adenosine slows it down, or "puts the brake on nerve transmission."[16]

Caffeine "increases the levels of acetylcholine, but, interferes with the transmission of adenosine." One might think this is wonderful of caffeine. But this is comparable, says Nedley, to driving a car without brakes. "This overstimulation of the brain causes unbalance of the mind, altering mood and behavior. So caffeine has been linked with anxiety, anxiety-neurosis, psychosis (a state where a person loses touch with reality), and even schizophrenia—the so-called 'split personality' disorder. Other researchers add to this list, caffeine-induced delirium and anorexia nervosa."[17, 18]

Not all studies agree with the following, but caffeine, in addition, has been associated with a variety of physical ailments, namely, high blood pressure; tachycardia (fast pulse); and high blood sugar, fats, and cholesterol. The results of some of these increases give people that "wake-up" feeling and make them feel they have extra energy. But there is evidence that instead of providing extra energy to the body, these chemicals actually "borrow from the body's energy reserves." Also, "hand coordination in performing fine detailed, complex tasks suffers."[19]

In the gastrointestinal tract, caffeine seems to interfere with the absorption of calcium, iron, and some of the B Vitamins (biotin and inositol), and increases the production of stomach acids.

"In the reproductive system, caffeine increases the risks of fibrocystic disease of the breast. As already mentioned, as a mutagenic substance, caffeine may increase bladder, pancreas, colon and breast cancer risks."[20, 21]

"Caffeine crosses the placenta, but as the fetus lacks the enzymes to break it down, it leads, in pregnant mothers who drink coffee, to stillbirths, premature births, slow fetal growth, decreased fetal birth weights, and birth defects."[22]

Caffeine has a diuretic effect on the kidneys and may aggravate asthmatic attacks.

Whether all studies agree or not, there is enough

to suggest abstinence. Without question, the best drink is pure water, as mentioned in chapter 3. This is especially important first thing in the morning, as the body gets dehydrated during the night.

Addiction—General View

Addiction, irrespective of the substance abused, has some common characteristics though expressed at different levels of intensity:

- Preoccupation with the substance: protecting the supply, planning for its use, etc.
- Loss of control: using more than planned and being unable to stop.
- Continued use despite adverse effects and circumstances: an alcoholic may have been told of liver damage but continues to drink; a smoker continues to smoke despite the presence of lung cancer.
- Depression: a common complication of addiction—and many patients are being treated with antidepressant medication instead of dealing with the addiction.
  - Inadequate and unsatisfactory interpersonal relationships: many social difficulties are frequent, with disturbed relationships in friendships, marriage, and employment.
- Hostility, with inappropriate expressions: rebellion, defying authority, anger, physical and verbal abuse.
- Denial of the above: a common occurrence—it blocks hope of treatment unless dealt with.

What are the chances for recovery from addiction? Although difficult, recovery is possible. But there must be a plan. Experts tell us that the basic plan of recovery for alcoholics or any substance abuser is:

- Realization that a problem exists: admitting powerlessness to "deal with" the problem. This may require "intervention," which is a process of gathering a group of concerned persons with the user and expertly pointing out the effects seen and the need for help.
- Seeking expert help.
- Accepting a program for recovery.
- Using that program in the life.

A successful program takes into consideration, among other things, treatment of withdrawal symptoms, education, reinforcement and support, a regulated, disciplined life, and last but not least, reliance on God as a loving Being and Father who will guide and comfort all who accept His invitation to "Come unto Me" (Matthew 11:28) and "Choose life" (Deuteronomy 30:19). For, "I am come," says Jesus, "that they might have life and have it more abundantly" (John 10:10). With total dependence upon God, victory comes when we claim the promise with Paul, "I can do all things through Christ which strengtheneth me" (Philippians 4:13).

Overweight

Earlier in this chapter, we defined *temperance* also as "moderate use of that which is good." This becomes significant in the area of nutrition—the avoidance of gluttony.

Overweight, or obesity, is a major problem in America and a contributing cause of most of our chronic illnesses. Overweight is implicated in the incidence of high blood pressure, heart disease, diabetes, cholecystitis, diverticulitis, and arthritis, as well as cancer of the breast, the endometrium, the kidneys, and the prostate. Studies have shown a correlation between the number of meals eaten in a day and the development of colon cancer. "Individuals who ate four meals a day had twice the incidence of colon and rectal cancer compared to those who ate two meals a day."[23]

In this respect, I would like to quote two interesting statements made ninety years apart:

- ■ 1994: "Carcinogens that cause only a small number of cancers in animals may cause several times more tumors in animals that are fed ad libitum rather than kept half starved."[24]

- ■ 1905: "Intemperate eating is often the cause of sickness, and what nature most needs is to be relieved of the undue burden that has been placed upon her. In many cases of sickness, the very best remedy is for the patient to fast for a meal or two, that the overworked organs of digestion may have an opportunity to rest. A fruit diet for a few days has often brought great relief to brain workers. Many times a short period of entire abstinence from food, followed by simple, moderate eating, has led to recovery through nature's own recuperative effort. An abstemious diet for a month or two would convince many sufferers that the path of self-denial is the path to health."[25]

Another fit example of science giving proof of accuracy, almost 100 years later, to a statement by Ellen G. White that some might have thought questionable!

The Frontal Lobe

"The path of self-denial is the path to health." Nowhere is this more true than in the area of pre- and extra-marital sexual conduct. Teen pregnancy and sexually transmitted diseases (STDs) are prevalent in society today and cause major social, psychological, medical, and spiritual problems. We need not recount the problems here. Our aim is to help point to the solution. Neil Nedley, in *Proof Positive*, devotes an entire chapter to the "frontal lobe" of the brain—the seat of our will power, reasoning, judgment, morality, and spirituality. He defines the frontal lobe as "the crown of the brain."

Nedley begins the chapter by describing Phineas P. Gage's accidental frontal lobotomy, which occurred in Vermont on September 13, 1848. Gage was the foreman in charge of blasting on railway construction in a mountainous area of Vermont—a devoted husband and father and pious and reverent churchgoer.

On that fateful morning, as the blasting charge was set off, instead of the "13-pound tamping iron, about one inch thick, and 3 feet long" going into the mountain "with the force of a missile, the iron came straight toward Phineas, entered under his left cheekbone, behind his left eye, through his brain, and then out again. The bar exited several inches behind his hairline after passing through Phineas' skull, scalp, and hair . . . and landed many yards away."

Gage did not die from the accident. He was "briefly stunned, but within a short time he regained full consciousness and was able to talk, and even walk with the assistance of his workers . .

. He survived . . . infections" in this preantibiotic era, "and made a nearly complete recovery, as far as his physical health was concerned. . . . There was just one major problem: he was no longer Phineas Gage."

Before the accident, he was known as a person with high morals, well-loved, responsible, and intelligent, and "the most efficient and capable foreman employed by the Ruthland and Burlington Railroad. After the accident, Gage was physically just as fit and mentally just as intelligent . . . His memory was just as good." However, "his moral decline was immediately evident. He became very emotional about things and would get angry quickly. . . . He lost interest in church and spiritual things . . . became irreverent and prone to profanity. He lost all respect for social customs and became totally irresponsible. He went from a prized employee to the unemployment rolls. His company dismissed him when he could no longer responsibly discharge his duties. . . . He ended up forsaking his wife and family, and joining a traveling circus. Phineas Gage's traumatic frontal lobotomy cost him his personality, his moral standards, and his commitment to family, church, and loved ones." Dr. John Harlow, his physician, stated that "the accident destroyed Gage's equilibrium or balance, so to speak, between his intellectual faculty and his animal propensities."

"Phineas died 13 years after the accident." To this day, his "skull along with the tamping iron . . . are housed in the Warren Anatomical Medical Museum at Harvard University."[26]

Nedley then, in detail, presents scientific data

which show that lifestyle habits can cause similar damage to our frontal lobe.

In addition to the drugs—prescription, nonprescription, illicit and the socially acceptable ones—we have just discussed (nicotine, alcohol, and caffeine), a diet with large consumption of refined sugar and flesh meat causes damage to our frontal lobe. Three additional habits in our lifestyle, because of their widespread use and great potential ill effects, demand our serious consideration: television, certain musical types, and transcendental, eastern-type meditation, or Yoga. It is thought provoking that the damage to the frontal lobe seems to be a "trance-like effect" akin to that caused by hypnotism. This is important, since hypnotism is used by some in the therapy of mental disorders and addiction, including nicotine addiction.

Hypnotism—Its significance

A word of explanation on hypnotism: "If brain waves were measured with an EEG (electroencephalogram) during the hypnotic state, we would see that the hypnotized person loses *beta* waves from the brain. Beta activity indicates sound thinking that involves dynamic frontal lobe activity. In the hypnotized state, however, an *alpha* brain pattern is operative, during which we do not critically analyze incoming information."[27]

Alpha waves are brain waves of a lower frequency than *beta* waves. In this state, an individual will record information and suggestions without interpretation and without frontal lobe filtering.

Television

Television has been dubbed the "home hypnotist." Jerry Mander explains that "TV watching fits the typical environment for hypnotism induction: a darkened room, a flickering light (TV set) as a single-minded focus, and freedom from all outside diversions." Then, not only does the content of what is seen on TV appear to influence the mind, the "very vehicle of TV itself is usually detrimental. The filming technique of a 'rapidly changing scene of reference' every 3 to 5 seconds in an average TV program, is in sharp contrast to how we normally view the world around us. In real life scenes, we change our perspective by voluntary action. TV's rapid change of reference contributes to its hypnotic effect."[28] Children watching their favorite shows were studied with EEGs. It was assumed that since it was their favorite shows, the children would be mentally involved with what they were viewing and would show a pattern of oscillating between alpha brain wave activity and beta. Instead, after just two or three minutes of the show, they sat back and stayed almost entirely in an alpha pattern. This means that while they were watching, they were "not reacting, nor orienting, nor focusing just spaced out."[29] Experts believe the same is true of adults.

Nedley presents in summary form seventeen harmful effects of TV watching. To name a few:

■ It produces a hypnotic effect, bypassing the frontal lobe.
■ It reduces interest in reading and learning.
■ It encourages poor lifestyle habits.
■ It weakens creativity.

■ It makes children especially more irritable.
■ It increases aggressiveness.
■ It accelerates sexual activity.
■ It steals time from family interaction.
■ It adversely affects spiritual pursuits.[30]

Music

What types of music cause damage to the frontal lobe?

"Music enters the brain through its emotional regions, which include the temporal lobe and limbic system. From there, some kinds of music tend to produce a frontal lobe response that influences the will, moral worth, and reasoning power. Other kinds of music will evoke very little, if any, frontal lobe response, but will produce a large emotional response with very little logical or moral interpretation."[31]

Studies have shown that the "syncopated" rock rhythm bypasses the frontal lobe and in addition causes structural damage to nerve cells in the temporal lobe itself—with abnormal branching and sprouting of nerve cells and disruption of messenger RNA, a chemical crucial to memory storage.[32] Thus, difficulty in learning and remembering ensues.

We mentioned at the beginning of the book that our bodies have a natural biological rhythm. Harmonic music synchronizes with this natural biological rhythm, whereas dysharmonic, syncopated music clashes with, or disrupts, this natural body rhythm. The detrimental results can include permanent learning difficulties. There is also evidence of actual atrophy (cell death) within the frontal lobe, with a resulting decrease in individual morality, self-worth, and reasoning power.[33]

Our children should be raised in an environment of harmonious types of hymns and symphonies. Research demonstrates that classical music helps college students learn spatial relationships in geometry.[34] Children three to five years of age scored significantly higher on the "object assembly" task of a puzzle—an exercise requiring frontal lobe function, after just eight months of group singing and keyboard lessons, compared to preschoolers who did not have music lessons.[35]

Musicians with perfect pitch were soundly exposed to music before age 7.[36]

My wife and I had the occasion of proving the value of classical music on the behavior of our 2- and 1-year-old "perfectly behaved" and "normal" grandchildren recently. We were both to be occupied with some home chores for a few minutes while babysitting. So my wife put on a tape of "Chopin for Children" and left them occupied with their toys. Within about three to five minutes, she excitedly called out to me into the family room. And—what a picture! Both these babies were sitting side by side on the sofa, quietly "reading" their picture books, which they had picked up themselves (we did not tell them to sit down, or read, or anything else). No question in our minds—they had both been influenced by the music, as far as we could determine. Obviously, we took pictures for posterity.

Transcendental (Eastern-type) meditation—Yoga

Eastern meditation, or yoga, is promoted for

stress control, but Dr. Freda Morris points out that in many cases it is really a technique of self-hypnosis.[37] For this reason, such meditation is potentially dangerous. The basic requirements are: a solitary focus—a single word, called a mantra, or a single shape or body part; a quiet environment; and a passive attitude, which Herbert Benson, a Harvard researcher, calls an "essential element."[38]

"If you connect stressed individuals to a biofeedback monitor (a stress-measuring device), whether they practice yoga or Eastern meditation, or pray to God, they will all very likely show significant stress reduction. However, only those who are praying still have their *reasoning powers fully intact.* The healthy, thinking beta brain waves will be present during prayer at the same time measurable stress reduction is occurring. Thus, communicating with God in prayer, with emphasis on actively reflecting on His Word, attempting to think His thoughts, sensing His presence, and knowing His will, thus, involving frontal lobe activity, addressing anxiety and fear without escapism relaxation techniques, provides a more balanced form of meditation."[39]

In addition, there is evidence of higher levels of stress hormone output and higher cardiovascular stress response in Yoga practitioners compared to nonpractitioners.[40, 41]

This seems consistent with work cited by Dr. Larry Dossey: "British psychologist Anne Manyande . . . and her colleagues examined blood levels of two stress hormones (adrenaline and cortisol) in patients just before surgery, in the recovery room, and on the 2 days following surgery. These stress hormones are believed to contribute to weight loss, fatigue, and impaired immune function surrounding surgery. They found that the stress hormone levels increased significantly only in those surgical patients who had formal relaxation training."[42] "Those that apparently dealt with their anxieties and fears without using escapism relaxation techniques did not show this rise in stress hormones."[43]

Says Nedley, in conclusion: "The chief message of this chapter . . . is to point out that, the most common causes of compromised frontal lobe function are improper lifestyle habits. . . . Many in our society today suffer the same tragic character defects evidenced by Phineas Gage after his traumatic frontal lobotomy. . . . Many of our most cherished habits give us short-term gratification, but silently rob us of that which is of inestimable value—who we are. Unknowingly, our habits today are impairing the performance of our frontal lobe today and tomorrow."[44]

So the ability to say "no" to nicotine, alcohol, caffeine, premarital and extramarital sex, MTV, or to that extra piece of sugary dessert, depends on a healthy and well-functioning frontal lobe. Could it be that stemming the tide of violence in our society and its betterment depends, as well, on each of us having a healthy and well-functioning frontal lobe?

It is within our power to exercise our minds and to provide our mental faculties the best possibility for development and expansion.

Notes:

1. NewStart: Lecture Notes on Temperance, Weimar Institute, Weimar, California.

2. Neil Nedley, M.D., *Proof Positive: How to Reliably Combat Disease and Achieve Optimal Health through Nutrition and Lifestyle* (Ardmore, Oklahoma: Quality Books, Inc. 1998), p. 2.
3. Ellen G. White, *Testimonies for the Church*, vol. 3 (Mountain View, Calif.: Pacific Press Publishing Association, 1948), p. 51.
4. Ellen G. White, *The Ministry of Healing* (Mountain View, Calif.: Pacific Press Publishing Association, 1905), p. 135.
5. Victor DeNoble, Ph.D., *Lectures and Personal Communications.*
6. Ibid.
7. Ellen G. White, *The Ministry of Healing* (Mountain View, Calif.: Pacific Press Publishing Association, 1905), pp. 327-329.
8. Vernon W. Foster, M.D., NewStar:, *New Health, New energy, New Joy!* (Santa Barbara: Woodbridge Press, 1988), p. 120.
9. Ibid.
10. Ibid.
11. U.S. Department of Health and Human Services. "Effects of Alcohol on Health and Body Systems." in Eighth Special Report to the U.S. Congress on Alcohol and Health. National Institutes of Health (NIH) Publication No.94-3699, Sep. 1993, pp. 171, 172.
12. Neil Nedley, M.D., *Proof Positive*, p. 432.
13. Ibid.
14. T.W. Rall, "Central Nervous System Stimulants (continued): The Methylxanthines." in *AG.*
15. Gilman and L.S. Goodman, et al., editors. *Goodman and Gilman's The Pharmacologic Basis of Therapeutics*, 7th edition (New York: MacMillan Publishing Company, 1985), p. 596.
16. S.I. Trevisanato, Y.I. Kim, "Tea and Health," *Nutrition Reviews* 58:1 Jan 1, 2000, 1-10.
17. Neil Nedley, M.D., *Proof Positive*, p. 269.
18. A. Kruger, "Chronic Psychiatric Patients' Use of Caffeine: Pharmacological Effects and Mechanisms," *Psycho. Rep.* 1996 Jun; 78(3 Pti): 915-923.
19. R.J. Edelman, S. Moxon, "The Effects of Caffeine on Psychological Functioning," *Nutr. Health*, 1985; 4(1) 29-36.
20. P.W. Curatolo, D. Robertson, "The Health Consequences of Caffeine," *Ann. Intern. Med.* 1983 May 98 (5Pt1) 641-653.
21. B. MacMahon, S. Yen, et al., "Coffee and Cancer of the Pancreas," *N. Engl. J. Med.* 1981, Mar 12; 304(11): 630-633.
22. D.A. Snowdon, R.L. Phillips, "Coffee Consumption and

risk of fatal cancers," *Am. J. Public Health*, 1984 Aug; 74(8): 820-823.

23. Neil Nedley, M.D., *Proof Positive*, p. 500.

24. S. Franceschi, C. LaVecchia, et al., "Meal frequency and risk of colorectal cancer," *Cancer Res.*, 1992, Jul 1; 52(13): 3589-3592.

25. Peter J. Morris and Ronald A. Malt, editors, *Oxford Textbook of Surgery* (Oxford: Oxford University Press, 1994), p. 2588.

26. Ellen G. White, *The Ministry of Healing* (Mountain View, Calif.: Pacific Press Publishing Association, 1905), p. 235.

27. Neil Nedley, M.D., *Proof Positive*, pp. 257, 258.

28. A. C. Guyton, *Textbook of Medical Physiology*, 8th edition (Philadelphia: W. B. Saunders Company, 1991), pp. 662, 663.

29. F. Morris, as quoted in J. Mander, *Four Arguments for the Elimination of Television* (New York: Quill, 1977), p. 208.

30. J. Mander, *Four Arguments*, p. 210.

31. Neil Nedley, *Proof Positive*, p. 287.

32. Ibid., 288.

33. G.M. Schreckenberg, H.H. Bird, "Neural Plasticity of MUS Musculus in Response to Disharmonic Sound," *The Bulletin*, New Jersey Academy of Science, 1987 Fall;32(2), 77-86, as quoted in Neil Nedley, M.D., Proof Positive, p. 288.

34. Ibid.

35. F.H. Rauscher, G. Shaw, K.N. Ky, "Listening to Mozart Enhances Spatial Temporal Reasoning: Towards a Neurophysiological Basis." *Neuroscience*, Letter 185, 1995, p. 46, as quoted by Neil Nedley, M.D. *Proof Positive*, p. 288.

36. F.H. Rauscher, G.L. Shaw, et al., "Music and Spatial Task Performance: A Causal Relationship," presented at the American Psychological Association 102nd Annual Convention in Los Angeles, California, August 12-16, 1994.

37. G. Schlaug, L Jancke, et al., "In vivo Evidence of Structural Brain Asymmetry in Musicians," *Science*, 1995 Feb 3: 267 (5198): 699-701, as quoted in Neil Nedley, M.D., *Proof Positive*, p. 289.

38. F. Morris, as quoted in J. Mander, *Four Arguments*, p. 208.

39. H. Benson, *The Relaxation Response* (New York: William Morrow and Company, Inc., 1975), p. 19.

40. Neil Nedley, M.D., *Proof Positive*, p. 279.

41. M.A. Wenger, B. K. Bagchi, "Studies of Autonomic Function in Practitioners of Yoga in India," *Behavioral Science*, 1961; 6:312-323.

129

42. A.E. Puente, I. Beiman, "The Effects of Behavior Therapy, Self-Relaxation, and Transcendental Meditation on Cardiovascular Stress Response," *J. Clin. Psychol.*, 1980 Jan 3(1): 291-295.
43. Bruce Bower, "Anxiety Before Surgery May Prove Helpful," *Science News* 141 (June 20, 1992): 406,407, as quoted in Larry Dossey, M.D. Healing Words, pp. 62, 63.
44. Neil Nedley, M.D., *Proof Positive*, pp. 258-297.

Chapter 9

"Don't you know that the Lord our God is the everlasting One? Haven't you heard that He always will be? He's the Creator of the universe! He never gets tired. He never gets weary. His understanding has no limits. He gives strength to those who are weak and energy to those who are weary. Even young men become weak and stumble and fall. But those who wait on the Lord and go to Him for help will have their strength renewed. They will soar like eagles. They will run and not be weary. They will walk and not faint" (Isaiah 40:28-31, *The Clear Word: An Expanded Paraphrase To Build Faith and Nurture Spiritual Growth*, by Jack J. Blanco)

"Let faith pierce the darkness. Walk with God in the dark as well as in the light, repeating the words, 'He is faithful that promised' (Heb. 10:23). Through the trial of our faith we shall be trained to trust in God."—Ellen G. White, *In Heavenly Places*, p. 89.

Trust in God

In this section we will discuss:

- Conceptualization of self-worth, based on one's belief of origin.
- Importance of mankind communing with God, the Creator.
- Through knowing God, mankind learns to trust Him.
- Despite good stewardship, mankind will die.

- Death: What is it? And what happens after death?
- The biblical proof of resurrection.
- Resurrection: The answer to what happens after death.
- A few meaningful, personal Bible promises.

Prescription No. 8:

Trust in God

God is a Friend. He has proven His love and friendship to us. He can be trusted. A relationship with God leads to happiness, peace, mental health, and security—both for the present and the future. The Bible is His "love letter" to us. Read it every day. That will foster trust in Him!

"Trust in God" is presented as the eighth and last of the "True Natural Remedies," but it is certainly not the least. In fact, we could by now say it is the most important. With some reflection on the previous presentations, we can see that it's been interwoven in all the other seven Natural Remedies.

God made us. Like the manufacturer of our automobile, He knows our body and what it needs to function properly. He supplies all our needs. He can be trusted.

Trust involves knowledge and acceptance of—belief and faith in—a person. Trust cannot develop unless there is an ongoing relationship. Relationship is nurtured through open communication.

God has taken the initiative to communicate with us. He speaks to us by His Word, the Bible, and by nature, His "lesson book." He has given us the tool and the means to speak to Him—prayer. Thus is established a two-way communication with God.

Without God taking the initiative, we would never know Him or anything about Him. He has chosen to reveal Himself to us.

In turn, our response to Him and to His initiative toward us is a matter of choice on our part. We choose to believe that He is what His Word says He is—the omnipotent, omnipresent, omniscient Creator of heaven and earth.

Our self-worth, I believe, is inherently connected to the concepts of our origin—two diametrically opposed concepts of our origin—expressed as the theory of creation, or the theory of evolution.

Just as the potter working with the clay does not need to explain to the clay who he is, the Bible simply begins with the words, "In the beginning God created the heaven and the earth" (Genesis 1:1) and then proceeds to describe the events of the first week of creation. Those events took place in a logical, intelligent, and purposeful manner—the events of one day supporting the next.

At the end of the sixth day, having pronounced man's creation "very good," God rested and made, blessed, and sanctified, the seventh day as a day of rest—the Sabbath.

As stated in an earlier chapter, I choose to be a Bible-believing, Christian creationist—among other reasons, because of the seven-day weekly cycle, which has no other basis for its existence than Genesis, chapter 1, and Genesis 2:1-3. Being a creationist provides me with "a worldview of a universe and human origins—my origin, from the hands of a Designer God."[1]

By contrast, Darwin, in 1859, borrowing the concept from Greek philosophers, devised an evolutionary development of species, published in his *Origin of Species*. The problem with belief in a molecular origin of man is that "it diminishes the potential of faith and tends to make man the supreme expression of the forces of the physical universe."[2]

Whether we admit it or not, we are dependent on the Bible for a knowledge of the early history of our world, of the creation of Adam and Eve, and of their fall. We accept the biblical history of the origin of life, or we are left to conjectures or fables.

Somehow, being "made a little lower than the angels," as David stated in Psalms 8:5, is more appealing to me than having, by chance, biologically evolved a little higher than the apes. More important, the evolution theory negates the fall of man from his high estate of being created in the image of God and of being redeemed by the death of Christ on the cross of Calvary. Man, in the process of evolution, has no need for a "plan of salvation;" has no need of a Savior. Self is enthroned; self-sufficiency, self-dependence, and self-righteousness motivate every action. Self-glorification fills the mind with pride. Pride worships the creature, not the Creator.

Pride belittles trust in any other but self. Pride negates faith in God and in His Word. Pride annuls communication with God. Pride stands in direct contrast with the Word of God, which invites us to commune with God, and His Son, Jesus Christ. Says 1 John 1:3: "That which we have seen and heard declare we unto you, that ye also may have fellowship with us: and truly our fellowship is with the Father, and with His Son Jesus Christ."

Of all the disciples, the apostle John knew and understood the benefits of communion with Jesus. From a "son of thunder," after three years of discipleship with Jesus, he became "John the beloved." He penned the new title "God is love" (1 John 4:8, 16). Such a realization comes only as we get to know God intimately. We feel safe and "welcome to His Throne," as writes Wesley L. Duewel in *Mighty Prevailing Prayer.*[3] In his introduction to prevailing prayer, Duewel comments, "God intends your praying to secure divine answers. Prayer is not just God's diversion to keep from being lonely. He delights in your fellowship. He always draws nearer when you pray."[4]

In total agreement, Ellen G. White says: "Prayer is the opening of the heart to God as to a friend."[5] Quoting Psalms 62:8—"Trust in Him at all times; ye people, pour out your heart before Him: God is a refuge for us"—she comments, "There is need of prayer—most earnest, fervent, agonizing prayer—such prayer as David offered when he exclaimed: as the hart panteth after the water brooks, so panteth my soul after Thee, O God."[6] We may therefore "come boldly," but humbly, "to the throne of grace"(Hebrews 4:16).

The Bible gives answers to basic human questions: Who am I? Where did I come from? Where am I going?

This book, thus far, has presented seven "natural" ways of combating illness and living longer. But we must realize, as stated so well by the late Vernon W. Foster, M.D., that "we cannot lifestyle ourselves into eternal life."[7] We live just so long—and we die. "Trust in God," the eighth Natural Remedy, assumes even greater significance as we face death.

What is death? What happens after death? These have been perplexing questions to humanity for a long time. The Bible explains what death is and does not leave us in the dark as to what happens after we die.

Jesus described death as a sleep from which the dead will be awakened by His call (John 11:11-14). Says John M. Fowler: "In so describing death as a sleep, Jesus was not simply waxing poetic. Nearly 66 times in 17 books, the Bible uses sleep as the figure of speech to describe death. And when Jesus authenticated such usage, He established two significant realities: the unconscious state of the dead and the certainty of their waking up either for judgment or for eternal life."[8] John 5:28, 29 states: "Marvel not at this: for the hour is coming, in the which all that are in the graves shall hear his voice, and shall come forth: they that have done good, unto the resurrection of life; and they that have done evil, unto the resurrection of damnation."

Christ's own resurrection and His raising of Lazarus give evidence both to the reality of death and to the power of Christ over death.

Says Isaiah: "Thy dead men shall live, together

with my dead body shall they arise. Awake and sing, ye that dwell in dust: for thy dew is as the dew of herbs, and the earth shall cast out the dead" (Isaiah 26:19). I like the New International Version (NIV) rendition of this verse: "Your dead will live; their bodies will rise. You who dwell in the dust, wake up and shout for joy. Your dew is like the dew of the morning, the earth will give birth to her dead."

Christ Himself says, "For my Father's will is that everyone who looks to the Son and believes in Him shall have eternal life, and I will raise him up at the last day" (John 6:40, NIV).

"Resurrection is not an easy doctrine to believe in. . . . Martha [Lazarus' sister] had a problem with obeying the command of Jesus to roll away the stone. Her fear of the stench rivaled her faith in the resurrection."[9]

Of all the world religions, Christianity only can claim an empty tomb! Paul, the apostle to the Gentiles, reminds us in Ephesians, chapters 1 and 2, that the same power which resurrected Christ from the grave will quicken us, who were "dead in trespasses and sins," will raise "us up together with Christ," and make "us sit together in heavenly places in Christ Jesus. . . . For we are His workmanship, created in Christ Jesus unto good works" (2:1-10). Paul is reminding us, as Christians, that we not only ought to die in Christ, but very important, also live in Christ, which will enable us to be resurrected in Him if we should die before He returns the second time. This power, therefore, quickens us to obey, not disobey, Him.

In 1 Corinthians 15, the greatest chapter, I

believe, on the resurrection in the Bible, Paul points out that the hope of the resurrection of the dead will be realized at the second advent of Jesus. "Behold," he says in verses 51-55, "I shew you a mystery; we shall not all sleep, but we shall all be changed, in a moment, in the twinkling of an eye, at the last trump: for the trumpet shall sound, and the dead shall be raised incorruptible, and we shall be changed. For this corruptible must put on incorruption, and this mortal must put on immortality. So when this corruptible shall have put on incorruption, and this mortal shall have put on immortality, then shall be brought to pass the saying that is written, death is swallowed up in victory. O death, where is thy sting? O grave, where is thy victory?"

I realize there are some seemingly contradictory passages in the Bible regarding the state of the dead. Philippians 1:21-24 may represent such a contradiction to some, where Paul states, "For to me to live is Christ, and to die is gain. But if I live in the flesh, this is the fruit of my labour: yet what I shall choose I wot not. For I am in a strait betwixt two, having a desire to depart, and to be with Christ; which is far better: Nevertheless to abide in the flesh is more needful for you."

It must be remembered that Paul had available to him Old Testament passages such as:

"For the living know that they shall die: but the dead know not anything, neither have they any more a reward; for the memory of them is forgotten. Also their love, and their hatred, and their envy, is now perished; neither have they any more a portion for ever in any thing that is done under the sun" (Ecclesiastes 9:5, 6).

"Put not your trust in princes, nor in the son of man, in whom there is no help. His breath goeth forth, he returneth to his earth; in that very day his thoughts perish" (Psalms 146:3, 4).

"The dead praise not the Lord, neither any that go down into silence" (Psalms 115:17).

"For in death there is no remembrance of thee: in the grave who shall give thee thanks?" (Psalms 6:5).

These passages must have helped him to conceptualize death, as a Christian. To Paul, dying in Christ—whether he spends one night in the grave or 2,000 years—the next voice he will hear will be that of Jesus welcoming him to life eternal. It seems that Paul, looking at the dying Christian, is comparing eternal life—which the Christian receives as he accepts Christ as his personal Savior—to a seed planted in the ground in the autumn, which then germinates in the spring. Says he: "Thou fool, that which thou sowest is not quickened, except it die: And that which thou sowest, thou sowest not that body that shall be, but bare grain, it may chance of wheat, or of some other grain: But God giveth it a body as it has pleased him, and to every seed his own body...So also is the resurrection of the dead. It is sown in corruption; it is raised in incorruption: it is sown in dishonour; it is raised in glory: it is sown in weakness; it is raised in power: it is sown a natural body; it is raised a spiritual body." (1 Corinthians 15:36-38, 42-44).

Having accepted Christ as personal Savior and Lord, if we are alive when He returns the second time, we will be changed in an instant. If we die before His second coming, we will be resurrected and given immortality then.

"Resurrection is, thus, God's answer to the problem of death. Christians must face death" not by denying it, but "by resting in the divine assurance of resurrection. There is no riddle or magic in this message. The Creator who brought the human being into existence can also resurrect that same being. It is as simple as that."[10]

In summary, God can be trusted. His Word, the Bible, can be trusted. Based on His sacrifice, the resurrection of Jesus Christ is, for all who accept Him as Savior and Lord, a bridge across the sleep of death, and it leads to a never-ending life of immortality, which—as Paul also states in 1 Corinthians 15:23—will be given to those "that are Christ's *at His coming*" (emphasis supplied).

We need not be perplexed about death!

Trusting God, as One worth our admiration and submission, will heal our spirit and most of our physical and emotional problems now. And if we should have to face death before the second coming of Jesus, we can do so with full confidence in the promise of the resurrection and the gift of immortality at His coming.

I believe it's fitting at the close of this chapter and of this book, to quote a few Bible promises that mean a lot to me:

- **Matthew 11:28**: "Come unto me all ye who labor and are heavy laden and I will give you rest."
- **Isaiah 26:3**: "Thou wilt keep him in perfect peace whose mind is stayed on thee."
- **John 14:27**: "My peace I give you . . . let not your heart be troubled."

- **Psalms 84:11**: "No good thing will He withhold from them that walk uprightly."
- **1 Peter 5:7**: "Casting all your care upon Him: for He careth for you."
- **Ephesians 3:20, 21** (my favorite): "Unto Him that is able to do exceeding abundantly above all that we ask or think, according to the power that worketh in us, to Him be glory in the church by Christ Jesus throughout all ages, world without end, Amen!"

Notes:

1. Vernon W. Foster, M.D., *NewStart:, New Health, New Energy, New Joy!* (Santa Barbara: Woodbridge Press, 1988), p. 242.
2. Ibid.
3. Wesley L. Duewel, *Mighty Prevailing Prayer* (Grand Rapids, Michigan: Zondervan Publishing House, 1990), p. 44.
4. Ibid., p. 13.
5. Ellen G. White, *Testimonies for the Church* (Mountain View, Calif.: Pacific Press Publishing Association, 1948), p. 533.
6. Ibid., p. 534.
7. Vernon W. Foster, M.D., *NewStart*, p. 240.
8. John M. Fowler, *The Cosmic Conflict Between Christ And Satan* (Nampa: Pacific Press Publishing Association, 2001), p. 87.
9. Ibid., p. 88.
10. Ibid., pp. 88, 89.

Postscript

I began by quoting two statements from *The Ministry of Healing*, which helped mold my thinking during my formative years and placed prayer prominently among my spiritual armaments as a young surgeon.

I thank God for the courage of being able—though at times timidly, but never forcibly—to offer to most of my patients the option of praying with them. I can count on one hand those who refused that option over the past twenty-nine years. It is wonderful to live and work in such an environment!

Events today in the medical field justify that decision of many years ago. The leading article in the May 2001 issue of *Reader's Digest* was entitled: "What doctors now know—the healing power of faith." The article went on to present and discuss the evidence.

It is important to point out that as scientists, especially in the West, we have disconnected science from spirituality, faith, and religion. It is noteworthy that scientific studies are responsible for bringing us back into line. Several examples were cited in the article. To name a few:

■ A nationwide study of 21,000 people from 1987 to 1995 found a seven-year difference in life expectancy between church-goers and non-church-goers.

■ Senior citizens who considered themselves religious had fewer health problems and functioned better than the nonreligious.

■ Patients who expressed comfort in their faith had a three times better chance of being alive six months after open heart surgery than those who did not find comfort in religion.

■ Patients in an intensive care cardiac unit who, without their knowledge, were prayed for, had fewer complications, shorter hospital stays, and survived longer, than those not prayed for.

Notwithstanding any flaws one may find in the design of these studies, the fact that they were carried out speaks loudly of courage on the part of the authors. They also demonstrate awareness of the need for a wholistic approach on our part as healing professionals. Such an approach must include the spiritual dimensions of our patients.

It is gratifying that at least one fourth of the medical schools today include some aspect of religious teaching in their curriculum. I believe the physicians of tomorrow, as a result, will be the better for it.